I0005651

Contents

Foreword

I have been fortunate enough to spend a lifetime in sport – from leading my first rugby team aged ten through to captaining Scotland and the British & Irish Lions. At an even younger age, I played golf with my family, and I now spend my spare time trying to keep my handicap in low single figures on the fairways of Gullane, Muirfield and St Andrews. Over the years, I've learnt a few things about pain, performance and longevity, and one of the most important lessons I've discovered is that you don't have to accept pain as the price of playing the game you love.

I've been lucky enough to have known Gavin Routledge for over thirty years. He's helped me navigate the wear and tear of rugby at the highest level and, more recently, the unique physical demands that golf places upon the body. His advice, insight and treatment have been nothing short of transformational – not just in managing pain but also in building the confidence to keep moving well, swinging freely and playing consistently at the desired level. That's why I'm so proud and happy to be writing this foreword to *Pain-free and Confident Golf*.

This book delivers what every golfer – whether amateur or elite – deserves: a clear, intelligent and practical approach to tackling one of the game's most persistent problems: lower back pain. It doesn't stop at short-term fixes. The six Essential Practices outlined in the book are designed to empower golfers to not only recover but to thrive – to move better, play better and enjoy the game for years to come. My goal is crystal clear: I want to be out there playing pain-free golf into my nineties. That might sound ambitious, but with the kind of knowledge and support found in this book, I have got to believe it's possible.

Whether you're recovering from injury, managing chronic discomfort or simply wanting to preserve your swing and your passion for the game, I can't recommend this book highly enough. It's thoughtful, it's science-based, it's the product of three decades of evolution in Gavin's personal and professional experience and, most importantly, it works.

Here's to golfing stronger, healthier and longer.

Gavin Hastings OBE
Former international rugby player and lifelong golfer

Introduction

'I just want to be able to keep playing golf into my nineties,' said Andy. There it was again. It was autumn 2023 and in the space of six weeks, this was the third of my golfing pals in their fifties saying pretty much exactly the same thing to me (Gavin and Gordon were the other two). They had all come in to consult me in the hope that I would give them a quick fix for their latest flare-up of lower back pain (LBP).

Here they were, all with a bit more time on their hands now their children had largely grown up (great – more golfing opportunities!), but there was a problem. They had more pain now than they'd had in their thirties, when they were playing more physical sports. Pain that was getting in the way of their favourite pastime. Pain that was undermining their enjoyment of their only remaining sport. Pain that meant their golf membership fees were looking like a shaky investment. Earlier that summer, Gordon had treated three of us to a round at Muirfield. There were two dodgy backs and a dodgy knee in that four-ball; fortunately, none of them were mine.

I'm aware it's a bit presumptuous to think you're going to make it into your nineties, but let's assume you do. What are your chances of still being able to play golf? One in four? One in five? Assuming you make it to that ripe old age, what is one of the biggest threats to you realising your golfing ambition? Yes, it's LBP.

LBP doesn't just affect men in their fifties. It affects us all, and it becomes more common with advancing age, plateauing in the over-seventies. I've written this book because I want my friends – and you – to be able to play as much golf as you'd like. I've had quite a bit of input from a range of golfers who have struggled with LBP and sciatica, including close friends.

What types of LBP is this book likely to help?

If you've been told that you have any of the below, this book will dispel many myths and misunderstandings. It will give you a framework on which you can build your own personalised plan for relief and long-term prevention of pain.

- Discs – prolapses, herniations, slipped, bulging, torn or degenerative
- Pelvic twist, misalignment or tilt
- Twisted spine
- Subluxations
- Weak or tight hamstrings, glutes or hip flexors
- A poor or weak core
- Glutes that don't fire
- Wear and tear
- Spondylosis or spondylitis
- Spondyloarthritis and more

If you have advanced degenerative changes with impingement on your lumbar or sacral nerves, the benefits to you will be lower, possibly marginal. If the phrase 'advanced degenerative changes with impingement' sounds like Greek to you, you almost certainly haven't got those severe problems. Happy days, because in that case there is good reason to hope.

What about me? Who am I?

I've been a practising osteopath for over thirty years, specialising in LBP and sciatica for most of that time. I have a Master's degree in The Clinical Management of Pain from The University of Edinburgh.

I've previously written two books on LBP – *The Back Book* with Gavin Hastings OBE in 1997 (HarperCollins) and twenty years later, a self-published book, *Active X Backs: An effective long-term solution for lower back pain.* (Don't bother with either – while they were good for their time, this one is way better and tailored to your needs as a golfer.)

I have also experienced more than my fair share of LBP and sciatica. I had seven years of episodic pain – from the age of nineteen to around twenty-six – until I finally worked out where I was going wrong (more on this later). That's when I wrote the first book with 'Big Gav', Gavin Hastings. He had quite a few problems with his lower back and my role was to try (along with other physical therapists and trainers) to ensure he was able to run out on the field on Saturdays, whether for club or country.

The aims of this book

There are a huge number of myths and misunderstandings about LBP and sciatica. As you will read, some of the diagnostic labels above are spurious, while others are barely relevant. I have found, through studying the research and experimenting in my own clinic, that relieving symptoms and preventing recurrence relies on some straightforward principles – I call them the Rules of Rehabilitation.

To me, steeped in professional and personal experience, the management of patients with LBP or sciatica is simple. That's right, I said 'simple' – don't believe for a moment that it's easy. I've been playing this game for over thirty years; I know where all the bunkers are, where people go wrong. I can coach you to become proficient in relieving and preventing LBP and sciatica. You can finally overcome this challenge.

We'll start by looking at how common LBP and sciatica are and introducing you to the Cliff of Pain in Part 1. Part 2 then focuses on Relief and we'll cover all the Relievers, Triggers, Aggravators and Risks of LBP. Part 3 focuses on understanding and I will talk you through the Pain Equation. Without this understanding, you will struggle to stick to the Prevention phase; if I simply gave you a long list (and, for some people, prevention is a long list), then at the first relapse you are likely to discard my whole approach as just another failed attempt. Understanding your persistent LBP will empower you to push ahead into prevention with enthusiasm and confidence. Part 4 will introduce you to the three Rules of Rehabilitation and the six Essential Practices, which will help you work towards a pain-free and confident future, before we cover a final few tips and our concluding thoughts. If you follow this book methodically, you will reach the nineteenth hole with your own personalised plan for both relief *and* prevention.

Yes, you could jump straight to the final part, but by playing the front nine before the back nine, you will end up with a plan that you understand and you're committed to – not just a dry plan with no context. If you don't understand why you're doing what you're doing and how to adapt to circumstances, as soon as you end up in the rough, you're likely to bin the whole approach. You have to understand why I'm suggesting these tactics; otherwise, you are playing the course blindfolded, swinging without any real idea what the hazards are in front of you. For your own sake, please work through this book methodically. I promise, it'll be worth it.

Let the dream become the reality

If the following dream scene resonates, this book is for you – the golfer who has tried it all yet refuses to accept that pain is an inevitable part of the game and of life; the golfer pursuing a long-term solution:

Imagine stepping onto the tee on the last day of a five-day golf trip, the sun warming your face, your body moving with ease as you swing your driver, confident that you'll complete the round without being hampered by your back.

This is not just a dream; it's a reality within your grasp. In this book, I'll guide you through the same transformative process that has helped countless

LBP and sciatica sufferers to reclaim their lives. Say goodbye to the cycle of temporary fixes and hello to a future where your back is your ally. Suffer less and play more. Discover the long-term prevention strategies that will keep you on the golf course and out of the chiropractor's office.

What this book doesn't offer

Before we get to the first tee, I'd like to tell you what this book doesn't offer and why.

This book does not offer a panacea – a one-size-fits-all quick-fix solution. There is no one solution for all, but there are principles that apply to everyone, which we'll cover in the three Rules of Rehabilitation and the six Essential Practices. It always amazes and disappoints me when self-help books just have a long list of actions without underlying principles. You need some anchors to hang on to because things *will* go wrong – that's part of the deal with long-term pain.

One more thing: there's a chapter in the book that I nearly didn't include. You might find it controversial or uncomfortable to read. If you're struggling with persistent pain, you have to exhaust all avenues – there isn't a 'magic key', but there are many contributing factors. Look out for that chapter – it's there because you need it, even though you might find it hard to swallow.

Being pain-free and confident

In choosing a title for this book, I surveyed over 100 golfers about their struggles and ambitions. 'Pain-free' and 'confident' kept coming up, and that's where the title came from – it resonated with me. For most of the last twenty years, I have been pain-free; for the last ten years, I have been confident. Confident that I know how to optimise my chances of staying pain-free and that – should pain happen – I will know why and I will know what to do about it. I'm also confident about staying fit and active into old age – something that I'm sure is also important to you.

You'll notice that I had ten years of being pain-free before I became confident. My aim is to dramatically shorten that time for you. Let's be honest, being pain-free all the time is just not realistic. Things happen, but they will be much less likely to happen to your back if you follow the guidance here. If they do happen, you will be confident that you can recover.

For example, a few years ago my mother-in-law asked if I could help move a large tub with a small tree planted in it. It meant moving it from the neighbour's garden, through their house, 20 yards between houses, through my mother-in-law's house and into her back garden. I'll spare you the details, but – being fearless (and overconfident) – I insisted on doing it myself. It was an awkward lift of a 40–45 kilogram circular tub that I could only get my arms partially around.

Yup, my back 'went', but it was fine seven days later. I wasn't worried; I knew what had done it and I knew I'd recover quickly. If you're as daft as me, you might hurt your back again. I can't guarantee that you'll be pain-free forever more, but by following this book, you'll be in a much better place than you are in now.

This is my promise to you: if you read this book from beginning to end, you will know everything you need to achieve a long-term solution to your lower back problem. If you act on what you learn, you can achieve it.

Safety first

I'm a clinician, and I would be letting both you and me down if we didn't cover safety at the outset of the book. Fewer than 0.5% of LBP sufferers have a serious underlying medical condition that needs medical management. If you answer 'yes' to any of the below 'red-flag' questions, this does not automatically mean that you need to see a doctor, but the more questions you answer 'yes' to, the more strongly I'd recommend that you do.

Red-flag questions

1. Compared with during your waking day, is your background pain worse when trying to sleep? (Not the sharper pain you get when you're turning over, just the constant type of ache.)

2. Have you lost any great amount of weight without meaning to over the last year?

3. Have you been diagnosed with cancer at any time?

4. Have you had lower back surgery in the last two years?

5. Do you have any numbness (lack of sensation) or pins and needles in your pelvic floor area (up between your upper thighs – the area you would sit on if on a saddle)?

6. Have you had any recent change in sexual function, eg loss of feeling, erection or ability to orgasm?

7. Do you have any difficulty urinating or defecating (using the toilet), eg trouble starting or stopping or not aware of your bladder filling up?

8. Have you suffered any significant trauma recently that in any way could impact on your lower back?

9. Have you been on a prolonged course of oral corticosteroids in the past or now?

10. Have you had a persistent high temperature recently?

Disclaimer

It is beyond the purposes of this book to discuss the possible implications of a 'yes' to each of the above questions, but it's my responsibility to flag up to you that sometimes (in fewer than 0.5% of LBP cases), there can be an underlying medical condition causing the pain. If you are struggling to get hold of a clinician to consult, we do provide video consultations. In authoring this book, I am not diagnosing the cause of your pain and you should consult a clinician if you have persistent LBP, with or without sciatica.

PART ONE
THE CLIFF OF PAIN

1
How Common Is Lower Back Pain?

L et's get a bit of perspective. Why are we here? Why is this a topic worth writing about – again? It's not just you that's suffering, is it? LBP is the talk of the locker room and the clubhouse. It is common and deeply frustrating for hundreds of millions of people around the planet – golfers and non-golfers alike – but how common is it?

LBP: The world's leading cause of disability

Every four years, a community of scientists comes together and publishes the Global Burden of Diseases (GBD) study. The measure they use to determine the impact of a disease or disorder is 'years lived with disability' (YLD).

Let's use Covid-19 as an example, which had a huge impact on our society. We all had to adapt to reduce the risk of catching it. Billions of pounds, dollars, yen and every currency in the world were invested in trying to solve the problem. In the first year of the Covid-19 pandemic, from April 2020 to March 2021, according to the GBD study there were 4.13 million YLD around the world due to Covid. That means that if you add up all the days of disability caused by Covid around the world in all the people infected, it equals 4.13 million years in that one year. Guess how many YLD were due to LBP in that same year?

There were 69 million YLD due to LBP between April 2020 and March 2021 (World Health Organization, 2020).

Perhaps not surprisingly, LBP has for decades been – and continues to be – the world's leading cause of disability. It won't kill you, but it can lead to years of problems. How much time and effort have you invested in trying to solve your LBP, compared with what you invested in responding to Covid-19?

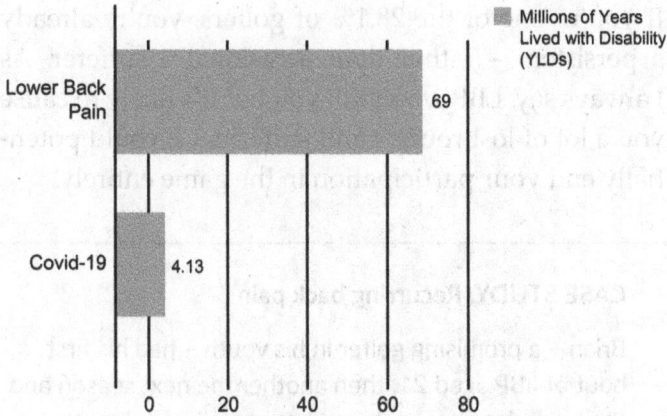

1.1 Global disability: April 2020–March 2021

How many of your golfing pals complain about their back after a round? According to Titleist Performance Institute (n.d.), 28.1% of all golfers complain of LBP after every round of golf.

Recovery and recurrences

It might look as though overcoming LBP is impossible, yet it isn't. There are millions of people who recover, but then they have another episode, don't they? Sixty-nine per cent of first-time sufferers have another episode within twelve months of the first episode resolving, according to da Silva *et al.* (2019). Recovery isn't so much the problem (at least when you first start suffering); the bigger problem is avoiding recurrences.

PAIN-FREE AND CONFIDENT GOLF

If you're one of the 28.1% of golfers, you're already a persistent – rather than occasional – sufferer. As I always say, LBP won't kill you but it's likely to cause you a lot of lost rounds and suffering. It could potentially end your participation in the game entirely.

CASE STUDY: Recurring back pain

Brian – a promising golfer in his youth – had his first bout of LBP aged 21, then another the next season and the following season. It just never really went away. Now in his forties, he can only manage one game a week with the help of anti-inflammatories.

Pain as a motivator

It's widely accepted that the evolutionary purpose of pain is to protect us. Think about it, if you put your hand in the fire, without pain you'd be likely to keep it there until it was burnt to a crisp. If you put your hand accidentally on the top of a hot cooker, it's likely that a reflex will cause you to pull it off before you even register pain, hopefully before any damage is done.

Pain can be useful. Consider the alternative: there is such a condition as congenital insensitivity to pain (CIP) (also known as congenital analgesia). There are a few gene mutations that can cause this. By early childhood, children with CIP have frequently suffered more injuries and infections than most (Schon *et al.*, 2018). A common problem is biting the tongue or the inside of the mouth. Even breaking a leg can be painless, leading the sufferer to continue to walk on it and do further damage. The inability to feel pain results in more rapid disability as joints degenerate through repeated injuries.

Much as pain is unpleasant, it does the job of motivating us to find out what is wrong and to change our behaviour. As a clinician specialising in LBP and sciatica for over three decades, I have seen the power of pain to motivate. My patients have been motivated to pay me – cumulatively – millions of pounds over this time. In the USA alone, medical costs from LBP are approaching $100Bn per annum, and economic costs are estimated to be around $600Bn. In the UK, the same figures are around £5Bn and £12Bn (*The Lancet*, 2023; Cook, 2024).

It's not all about the swing

It's worth acknowledging that LBP is common among non-golfers. When I reviewed the evidence in 2014, the indicators were that 23% of the adult population – more than one in five people – had persistent LBP. The research doesn't provide an exact comparison of golfers to non-golfers. As cited above, Titleist's figure was that 28.1% of golfer's report pain after every round. Now, if you assume (which you should never do in the world of medical research) that all those golfers were playing golf fairly frequently, then you might conclude that 28% of golfers have persistent LBP. Compared with 23% of the population as a whole, it's not a huge difference. Therefore, it's not all about the swing!

Simple fact: you do have to swing to move the ball closer to the hole. Is it the golf swing that's the cause of LBP, or other aspects of life, or both? If golf is contributing, do you have to swing in such a way that your lower back gets sore? We'll cover this and more later in the book. In the meantime, let me tell you the story of how I developed the first framework, the Cliff of Pain, which is going to give you a powerful new way to think about your LBP.

Summary

- LBP is the world's leading cause of disability.

- Overcoming recurring LBP is possible.

- Pain can be a useful motivator.

- LBP is common among non-golfers – it's not all about the swing.

2
Understanding
The Cliff Of Pain

I n this chapter, you will learn the first framework
that will enable you to fully understand why – so
far – you've been unable to achieve a lasting solution.
It's a simple but powerful model that you can apply
immediately. I've been using it for thirty years in clinical practice, and I wrote about it in my first book on
LBP in 1997.

My own Cliff of Pain

It was late February 1992 and autumn was coming.
My girlfriend and I had been driving through the
South Island of New Zealand for the previous two
weeks. We had driven for a few hours most days and
then spent the afternoons and evenings enjoying each

new destination. We arrived in Dunedin, where a friend had offered to put us up for a couple of nights.

After a wander through the town, we found ourselves on the beach, about fifteen minutes' walk from our friend's apartment. A big black dog came bounding up to us, with a stick in his mouth, which he dropped at my feet. I love dogs. I bent down to pick the stick up and that's when it happened.

That moment changed the course of my life. I'd had similar experiences before – locking up my bike, picking a glass up from a table, stooping to shave – but this episode turned out to be the straw that broke the camel's back. It finally moved me from sufferer to conqueror, from student to master.

As I stooped to pick the stick up – wham! A spasm of pain shot across my lower back. I dropped to my knees. It was pure agony. My girlfriend had seen it all before, of course. She helped me back to the apartment, which – remember – was only fifteen minutes' walk away. It took us an hour.

Our friend was a student at the University of Otago. Like many young men, cleanliness wasn't high on his priority list. His living room carpet needed a good clean; it was brown and it had lots of flecks of 'stuff' in it. I don't know what the stuff was – maybe old bits of food – I didn't care to inspect it. I knew it was a mess because I spent the next three days and nights lying on that dirty brown carpet in his living room. It was agony to move, but after ten minutes of lying still in any position the pain escalated to the point I felt I had to move, which shot spasms of pain all across my lower back. By day two, I had sciatic pain too. It was miserable. To this day, I have no memory of how my girlfriend spent that time. I was in my own world of suffering.

I'd been here before, but I had recovered previously, then it had happened again. I had found relief, but I couldn't seem to prevent the pain from coming back.

Over those days of suffering, I had time to reflect that the hard truth was that all the things I'd found to relieve my pain didn't stop it from recurring. I needed a model for planning my route to a long-term solution. That's what came to me when I had recovered sufficiently to continue on our journey. Lying back, fully reclined in the passenger seat, watching the cloudy sky zoom past the window as my girlfriend drove us home to the North Island of New Zealand, this idea came to me.

The long-term solution

If you've been in agony, you'll know how keen we are to find relief. I had been focused on relief – pain is a great motivator for that. Having achieved relief, I had reverted to my old habits and then had another flare-up. The model that came to me, and the one I recommend to you (if you're looking for a long-term solution), is called the Cliff of Pain™.

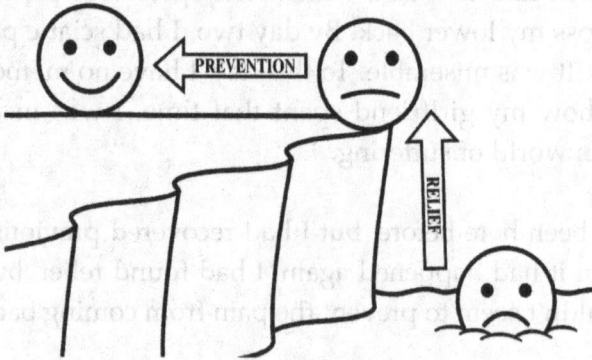

2.1 The Cliff of Pain: Relief and prevention

Most of us find ways of relieving our pain but they don't stop the pain from flaring up again. That's because relief and prevention are two different processes, which is reflected in Figure 2.1. Relief gets you out of the Sea of Suffering and back onto the cliff top, while prevention gets you right back from the edge. Two stages: relief and then prevention. I'll unpack both of these as you progress through the book, but let's expand on the Cliff of Pain model for now.

Some people have said the cliff should be the other way round, because you want to progress from left to right, but to reflect your journey up to this point we have to show how you got to be in the Sea of

Suffering. In reality, your journey begins when you're feeling fine, over on the far left. As most of the readers in the world work this way – from left to right – that's how I've laid it out.

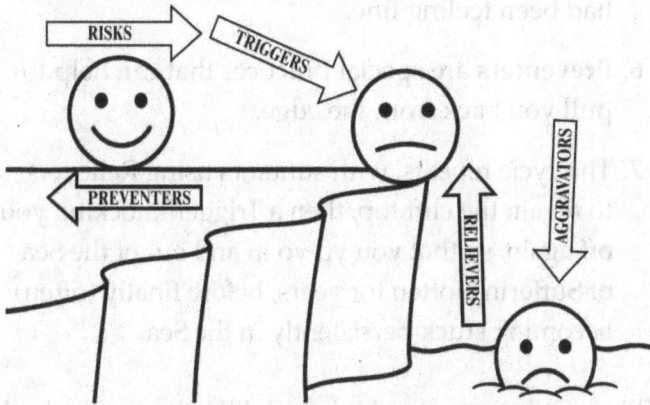

2.2 Expanding on the Cliff of Pain model

Here's how the journey unfolds:

1. **Risks** silently push you closer to the edge.

2. **Triggers** knock you off into the Sea of Suffering. This may cause sudden obvious onsets of pain, but it may be more gradual. (I had many Triggers over my years of suffering – most of them involved bending forwards, like picking up the dog's stick.)

3. When you're in the Sea of Suffering, **Aggravators** are things that make your pain feel worse. (Sitting was the most obvious one for me.)

4. **Relievers** help you regain the cliff top. (Manual therapy usually worked for me, and I evolved a number of exercises.)

5. **Triggers** knock you off the cliff again when you had been feeling fine.

6. **Preventers** are special practices that can help to pull you back from the edge.

7. The cycle repeats, with sufferers using Relievers to regain the cliff top, then a Trigger knocking you off again, so that you yo-yo in and out of the Sea of Suffering, often for years, before finally (often) becoming stuck persistently in the Sea.

This is an important point, which I'll keep coming back to through the pages of this book. As you can see from our model, Relievers – including relieving exercises (different to Preventer exercises), medication, relaxation, meditation and manipulation/massage – only help you regain the cliff top. They don't help to pull you back from the edge of another fall. We'll unpack all of the Risks, Triggers, Aggravators, Relievers and Preventers as you progress through the book.

TRY IT YOURSELF

Try drawing your personal Cliff of Pain and adding in your own Triggers, Aggravators, Relievers, Preventers and Risks as you work your way through the book.

Summary

- The Cliff of Pain model differentiates between short-term relief and long-term prevention of pain.

- Triggers and Aggravators play significant roles in falling into and staying in the Sea of Suffering.

- Relievers help to regain comfort temporarily, but Preventers are necessary for lasting relief from pain.

- Recognised Relievers include: exercises, medication, relaxation, meditation and manual therapy.

PART TWO
RELIEF

3
Relievers

I n this chapter we will cover the recognised Relievers for LBP and sciatica. I didn't see it this way at the time, but perhaps the most valuable – and certainly formative – part of my four years as an osteopathic student was having LBP and sciatica for most of that time. When studying to be an osteopath, I had another incident that left a mark on my belief system from early on. Let me take you back three years before my New Zealand episode.

In London, at the British School of Osteopathy (now the University College of Osteopathy) in 1989, one of my clinical tutors said something to me that has shaped my approach ever since. Dr Peter Randall was a white-haired man in his fifties, who seemed – to a twenty year old – to be as wise as Yoda. He had a twinkle in his eye and enjoyed sharing his wisdom.

I don't know whether he said this to all of his osteopathic students; I suspect not. I was a confident (hopefully not overconfident) student and I had just presented a case history to Doc Randall (when a clinician gives the outline of the patient's story) for my first new patient of the morning. I gave my working hypothesis of what may be wrong with this man, then the next step was for me to go and examine him, refine my thinking and progress to treatment. As I walked away from our discussion, Doc Randall called after me, 'Remember, Gavin. Many of your patients will get better…' – he paused for dramatic effect – '…despite what you do to them.'

I was pretty puzzled by what he'd said but was busy thinking about my patient. As I mulled this over later, I became increasingly annoyed. How could he say such a thing? Was he questioning the value of the profession I was working so hard to join? Or was he simply reminding me that I – and other clinicians – might be wrong, and that even when we're wrong, many people will still get better?

Nature helps to heal

Our bodies are changing all the time. There's a principle here called homeostasis, in which your body is constantly attempting to return to an optimal state. Why? In order to keep you alive. It wouldn't be much good if your body didn't attempt to heal itself. You'd have to go and get stitched up for the smallest of cuts. In health, when you cut yourself, the blood clots; this is a visible homeostatic mechanism.

Inflammation is a homeostatic mechanism too – it's an important part of healing. In fact, it's the first stage. Admittedly, in some people inflammation gets out of hand and becomes damaging rather than beneficial, eg in cases of rheumatoid arthritis, ulcerative colitis and systemic lupus erythematosus. This is rarely the case in LBP.

Muscular strains heal pretty quickly; usually in two to four weeks in healthy young adults. Intervertebral discs tend to be one of the slowest tissues to heal (they don't have a direct blood supply, see Chapter 4). If you have a prolapsed disc, take heart; research shows that they heal too. If you do the right things, many discs can recover over several weeks to a few months. In fact, the bulge often varies in size – even within a day.

CASE STUDY: Disc prolapse recovery

Angus had been in pain for three months when he first consulted me. He was stooped forward and tilted to one side. The MRI clearly showed a sizeable disc prolapse at L4L5, which matched his symptoms of LBP and sciatica. He had a surgical date booked.

Following the Rules of Rehabilitation (coming later), his pain improved significantly over the next eight weeks. Three months after that, he was skiing in the French Alps. He was happy to have avoided the surgeon's knife (and his fee).

Inflammation can be your friend

Inflammation helps you to heal; in fact, you're unlikely to heal well without it. It's vital that inflammation happens. The second stage of healing (scar tissue formation) kicks in as the inflammatory phase completes.

There is some evidence now that taking anti-inflammatory drugs after injury can delay healing of bone, tendon and the junction between bone and tendon (Su and O'Connor, 2013). Most of these studies have been conducted in animals, but the mechanism is clearly there for non-steroidal anti-inflammatory drugs (NSAIDs) to slow up healing. Remember to consult your physician before making any changes to your medication.

Inflammation is your body's way of bringing in all the ingredients required to repair damage, and to fight infection if it's there. Unfortunately, inflammation hurts. It sensitises your nociceptors (pain nerves – see Chapter 6), making them more likely to 'fire'.

You may have a constant ache if you're inflamed. It's usually worse in the mornings because the inflammation builds up while you lie still. Osteoarthritic knees are usually stiff and sore to get moving after you've been sitting for a while – that's the build-up of inflammation.

If you'd like me to take you through the whole Relief phase in a free short video and audio programme online, visit https://golf.painfreeandconfident.com/book-reader or just scan the QR code below:

Recommended Relievers

Let's move on to cover some recommended Relievers. Does it matter which Relievers you use? Probably not, so long as they do what it says on the tin (that is to say, if it works for you, great). If you've found ways of relieving your pain, then that's fine with me. Some of the ways recommended in the international clinical guidelines are covered in the next few pages.

Medication

It's an obvious place to start and one that you've probably tried, but which pills and potions actually work for LBP and sciatica?

Before diving in, I have a simple question for you: Do you think medication speeds up tissue healing?

No, it doesn't speed up healing; all it does is mask the symptoms. Anti-inflammatories don't speed up the healing either; in fact, they can slow down the rate of healing of certain tissues.

I am not saying that you shouldn't take them – you should consult your doctor about the pros and cons of medication and then make an informed decision – all I can tell you is what I do. I have used pain-relieving medication if the pain was significantly reducing the quantity and/or quality of my sleep (as we'll cover in Chapter 12, sleep is important). I don't use medication to do more of what would be painful without it. Why? Because pain is there to warn you when to stop. If you mask it and carry on, you are breaking the first Rule of Rehabilitation (coming up in Chapter 9).

NSAIDs are recommended in many countries for LBP. If these don't relieve the pain, opioid medications are frequently recommended in the short term, often combined with paracetamol or acetaminophen.

Opioid medications should only be used for a few weeks at most. They can lead to significant side effects and are addictive for many people. The opioid crisis is huge in the USA and in many other countries. A lot of this opioid addiction has been as a result of people trying to deal with persistent pain. If you're using pain relief in the short term, the simplest approach is to take the NSAIDs as prescribed and to supplement with paracetamol or acetaminophen in between.

As long ago as 2013, a review of the evidence for opioid treatment of chronic LBP concluded that there is low to moderate evidence that they are helpful in the short term, ie in the Relief phase (Chaparro *et al.*, 2013). There is no evidence of efficacy (how effective they are) or safety in their use for more than a few weeks.

In short, if you use opiates in the short term they may reduce your pain. If you take them for more than a couple of weeks, they become less effective and you are at risk of addiction. The risk–return is not worth it.

TOP TIP

You should consult your physician before making any changes to your use of medication.

Another type of drug often used for persistent pain is the antidepressant group. Mood and pain have common pathways in the brain, so antidepressants are

PAIN-FREE AND CONFIDENT GOLF

often used for persistent pain. Some drugs are better for relieving neurogenic sciatica (see Chapter 6). These must be prescribed in the UK and many other countries, and – whether prescribed or not – you should always discuss with your doctor or pharmacist how best to use them. Amitriptyline and gabapentin are examples of this type of drug. These drugs are rarely prescribed for LBP – just for types of sciatica.

Manual therapy

Many countries recommend chiropractic, osteopathy and physical therapy (including massage) for LBP. Some countries only do so for short-term pain, others for longer-term pain. All countries recommend using manual therapy in combination with other interventions (most commonly exercise), rather than depending on it exclusively.

Acupuncture

Some countries say yes, others say no.

Hot/cold therapy

Again, there are mixed views on this. If you have clearly injured your lower back, for example in a heavy lift or trauma, then most authorities promote ice-packing for the first forty-eight hours.

TOP TIP

Wrap your ice pack in a thin tea towel so you don't burn the skin, and hold on for twenty-five minutes.

After the first two days, heat tends to be more beneficial. Try to work out which works best for you – if either.

TENS

Transcutaneous electro-neural stimulation (TENS) is rarely recommended, but it helps some people some of the time – especially those with sciatica.

Movement and exercise

This is one of the strongest levers you can pull.

Which exercises? A quick internet search gave me around 220 million results in 0.3 seconds. A few of them will be articles and videos I have published on this subject. I have included images of exercises in previous books, but words and pictures are nowhere near as good as video at demonstrating exercises.

Please make use of the free Rapid Relief Plan by scanning the QR code below or visiting https://golf.pain-freeandconfident.com/book-reader. It includes all the exercises you need, tailored to you and providing lots of guidance on Relief. If you're in Scotland – the home of golf – near Edinburgh or East Lothian, we can package this up with manual therapy, so you can achieve more rapid relief.

Mix it up and stay busy

We'll be deepening your understanding of pain with The Pain Equation in Chapter 6. When you have that understanding, you'll see why this is important. Breaking up your activities into small chunks, varying what you do and staying busy is key during the Relief phase.

When I graduated in the early 1990s, many doctors were still recommending that LBP sufferers have two weeks of bed rest. This was terrible advice for the vast majority of people. Don't do that. Far better to stay as active as you can, while following the first two Rules of Rehabilitation (see Chapters 9 and 12). Mixing it up is difficult when you want to play eighteen holes of golf. Guess what, you might be better to play nine, or even five or six in the early stages of Relief.

The problem with Relief

Overtreatment for LBP

If you live in a city of more than half a million people in Europe, North America or Australasia, there are probably more than 100 healthcare professionals in your city who treat people with LBP and sciatica. Osteos, chiros, physios (PTs in the USA), massage therapists, sports therapists, acupuncturists and all sorts of other therapists. They will all claim to be able to help, and many of them can. Up to a point. Manual therapy, in particular, is recommended for short-term LBP and sciatica. Most countries who have published clinical guidelines on LBP and sciatica recommend manual therapy in its different forms.

Note I said 'short term'. A few of these countries include a much less enthusiastic recommendation for manual therapy for long-term LBP/sciatica, but *only* when it's to supplement the more highly recommended interventions (more on those later).

Here's the problem. Because manual (and other) therapies are effective at providing relief, many people think that more of the same thing has to be even better and will ultimately solve the problem. If you feel 50% better after five massage appointments, you'd be forgiven for thinking that it's only a matter of a few more treatments to solve the problem forever. While this might seem obvious to some, it is completely wrong.

It's like saying, 'That soup, salad and sandwich took away my hunger pangs. If I eat several helpings, then I shall never be hungry again.'

CASE STUDY: Chiropractic treatment vs. exercise

Jake estimated that over the last five years he'd had in excess of 200 chiropractic visits. Initially, he'd felt better after appointments, but lately treatment didn't seem to help at all. His back pain had been building over the last six months to the point that golf had become impossible.

Examination revealed that he had instability in his L3L4 joint, so I suggested he stop having manipulative treatments and instead follow an exercise regime. Quite quickly, his back settled down to the point he could play once a week again. That gave us something to build on.

The perils of painkillers

Painkilling medications are also tempting; however, their effects wear off and they hold another set of perils too. Some are addictive, some cause damaging side effects and some can do both. The USA has a higher opiate crisis than other countries; however, it's present to some extent in many countries. In many cases of addiction, the opiates were originally prescribed for LBP or sciatica.

There's a saying in marketing: 'It's easier to sell a painkiller than a vitamin.' Hence the size of the LBP industry. Nearly all parties are selling painkillers and – from a business perspective – quite rightly. I do this too. I have had clinics in Scotland for over thirty years and have a long history in providing relief for golfers prone to back pain.

CASE STUDY: VIP treatment

Way back in 1995, I was asked to go up to Gleneagles (an hour's drive from Edinburgh) to treat Bob Hope. He was ninety-two by then and was playing golf daily on his three-day visit to Scotland. His aide wanted him to have daily manual therapy, and I was the man for the job. This is something he had at home and whenever travelling. It helped to relieve his pain and free him up for his beloved golf.

Relief and prevention are different processes

The biggest problem with Relievers – whether they be drugs, manual therapy, acupuncture, exercise or whatever – is that they only provide relief. That sentence may not make sense to you. What's wrong with relief? We all want relief, right?

Depending on which dictionary you use, there are variations on the definition of relief. Here's one from Merriam Webster: Relief – 'removal or lightening of something oppressive, painful, or distressing.' Sounds good, right? We all want that. Here's the definition of another word: Prevention – 'the act of preventing or hindering.'

Those are clearly different things, aren't they? We're coming full circle back to the Cliff of Pain – often, this is a light-bulb moment for people, just as it was for me lying back in the passenger seat in New Zealand. I'm only going to make this point once more before leaving it alone – I don't want to be condescending. If I were speaking it to you, I would do so slowly, to emphasise the point. Please read the next sentence to yourself slowly, pausing between the words:

Relief – and – prevention – are – totally – different – processes.

It is super-important that you understand and act on this. Put simply, relief and prevention are different – that which gets you relief will not prevent recurrence. More than that, I have found in clinical practice that pursuing relieving practices is so tempting and gratifying that it distracts sufferers from the longer-term goal – achieving prevention.

You may think that seeing your chiropractor monthly is preventing LBP. Personally, I doubt it. As I said earlier, it's like eating when you're hungry – it will relieve the symptom for a while, but it will not prevent it from recurring. Remember Doc Randall's insight: 'Many patients will get better, *despite* what you do to them.'

Unfortunately, pain is a tremendous motivator. When you're in pain, you will pursue relief, but once the pain has gone, your motivation goes with it, so you never fully commit to the prevention process and you revert to your old habits in the long term. It's human nature to conserve energy and other resources for when we need them. It's a big problem for humans; we might think about long-term goals but we are motivated and act in the short term.

Summary

- Inflammation is a necessary part of healing.

- Seeing a physical therapist regularly may not prevent pain recurrence.

- Pain is a significant motivator, leading to a short-term relief focus.

- Motivation for prevention often dissipates with pain relief.

- Humans tend to conserve resources for immediate needs.

- Long-term goals are often overshadowed by short-term actions.

4
Triggers And Aggravators

I n this chapter we'll take a high-level look at Triggers and Aggravators. We'll define each term and cover what to do about them.

Triggers

Triggers knock you off the edge. They move you from no pain to pain. Sometimes they are obvious and sometimes they are not.

One of the most common phrases I hear in clinic is, 'All I was doing was....'. When I hear it, I know we've found a Trigger. It's not really the cause. It's just the thing that pushed you off the edge. For many golf-ers, the golf swing can be a Trigger. Or bending over to put the tee in the ground. Or getting your ball out of the hole. Picking up the stick to throw for that dog in Dunedin was my Trigger; my back was already primed to 'go'.

If you're not sure what yours are, think about your Aggravators and consider them as possible Trigger suspects.

Aggravators

Aggravators make the pain you already have feel worse. The movements that aggravate your pain will form part of your Functional Assessment (covered in Chapter 9 and in the Rapid Relief Plan – see Chapter 3 for QR code). Dealing with Triggers and Aggravators is an important part of getting better. It is addressed in the first Rule of Rehabilitation and in the first of the six Essential Practices (both of which you will also read about in Chapter 9).

If you're following my process so far, you'll have guessed that you must reduce your Aggravators in the short term. If you don't reduce them, your return to the cliff top will be slowed, and possibly prevented entirely. In short, if you keep doing Aggravators, you may be stuck in the Sea of Suffering for a long time.

Move it, don't stretch it

As an example of an Aggravator, let's consider stretching. Stretching exercises are widely recommended by many in the profession. There's been a long-held belief by many (clinicians included) that stretching is good for you, but guess what? Stretching might not be good for your back. It might be good for someone else's back, but it might not be for yours.

CASE STUDY: Stopping stretching

Adrienne had been doing stretching exercises recommended by her sports physio for the last six months. It felt good when she did them. She felt she was making a difference by doing something to help herself.

Quite often, she had more LBP the morning after doing her stretches. She certainly hadn't been making progress; if anything, her pain was slowly worsening.

Within two days of stopping the stretching, her pain reduced by 50%.

For a significant percentage of the golfers I see, stretching feels good but it's actually aggravating their problem. The simple truth is that there is no one-size-fits-all approach. Your back problem is different to the next person's. Any sweeping advice on what's good and what isn't is an oversimplification.

Why stretching could be holding you back

In spinal mechanics, instability refers to a joint – or more than one joint – that is poorly controlled by the muscles operating over it. You could think of it as a wobbly joint among stiffer joints. This can be a problem.

Your spine consists of a series of blocks (vertebrae) linked together (joints). Over time – or perhaps due to trauma – one of those joints becomes more mobile than its neighbours. When you bend and move (eg swing a golf club) you're in danger of overworking that joint because the loosest one will move first. If you do overwork it (strain it), it'll get sore.

There are tests for instability that we routinely use in our clinic. Sorry, it's impossible to do to yourself. Symptoms that suggest you have an unstable joint in your lower back are sharp pains turning over in bed or getting out of a chair. Unfortunately, these symptoms don't guarantee that you have instability, but without these symptoms it's less likely that you have it. Another way to test for it yourself is bracing (we'll cover that in Chapter 12).

What does this have to do with stretching? Well, if you have lumbar spine instability, you shouldn't be stretching it. Think about it. If one of your joints moves more readily than the others, when you stretch, that joint will move first. There's a danger you are just perpetuating the instability and that's a bad idea.

> **TRY IT YOURSELF**
>
> If you've been following a particular exercise regime for a while and you're not improving, consider stopping it. At worst, you'll gain some time; at best, you may feel better for not doing those exercises.

Stretching discs and picking scabs

Here's another reason not to stretch. If you have a tear in one of your discs (that's right; they don't 'slip', they tear – more on this in Chapter 7), that tear needs to heal by the formation of scar tissue. If you stretch it too early or too much, you will re-tear the scar tissue. That kicks you right back to the early stages of healing, ie inflammation, meaning you're in more pain again and you've delayed healing.

I liken this to picking a scab before it's ready to fall off. Discs are slow to heal because you reach maturity without them having a direct blood supply (see Chapter 4). Studies show that they only get a direct blood supply (in some people) after you've injured them – and that's a small blood vessel. With or without this small blood vessel, they are slow to heal. Stretching the scar tissue before it's well formed is a good way to delay healing or prevent it entirely. We'll get into rehabbing discs in Chapter 7.

Stretching could be bad for your back, but then again it might not be. Which exercises are right for you should be based on your Functional Assessment (see Chapter 9), which is different to a diagnosis. You can get your Functional Assessment and the appropriate exercises in the Rapid Relief Plan (see Chapter 3 for QR code).

Is it the swing?

The golf swing exerts significant forces on your lower back. According to Hosea, Gatt and Galli (2010), a full swing can result in peak loads in your lower back of up to eight times your total body weight. There are multiple directions of force, including sideways sliding, sideways bending, downward compression and back-to-front shearing.

That's quite a lot of force, isn't it? In fact, if you were looking for an ideal way to injure your lower back it would be something that you do repeatedly, that is a vigorous movement, done with momentum, and combines a number of different movements. Sounds like a reasonable description of golf, doesn't it? That's quite a combination. If you're focused on maximising clubhead speed, you're also likely to be increasing forces generated through the spine.

If you're trying to hit the ball as far as you can, you're probably generating as much force as you can muster. Perhaps a useful question might be: Do you have to swing in such a way that your lower back gets sore?

There's a good chance you've tried shortening your backswing. We've all done that, haven't we? Reducing the amplitude reduces the forces on your lower back.

You could try slowing your swing down too, as speed is related to force. You probably don't want to do that, because then you'll be known as a short-hitter. So embarrassing. What if it meant you were pain-free, and by doing that – at least in the short term – you were able to keep playing golf?

I'm guessing you're not driving the ball over 300 yards (although some of my patients do). Losing 30 yards off the tee isn't going to ruin your score, especially if it improves your accuracy. Admittedly, at the top level, those who drive furthest make the most money. Are you playing at that level or are you just trying to keep playing?

What else could you do to swing in such a way that your lower back doesn't get sore? Well, you could try swinging differently. Wouldn't that mess up your game? Maybe, but then your pain probably messes up your game anyway. Left for long enough, the pain may jeopardise your ability to play at all.

A little bit more on swing technique. It's estimated that the classic swing exerts less load on the lower back than the modern X-Factor Swing. Plus, there are other swing options for reducing load (we'll get into that in Chapter 15).

TRY IT YOURSELF

Try shortening your backswing (I know it's obvious, but have you tried it?). Turning your lead foot out can also reduce the load on your lower back by enabling your hips to rotate through more easily.

Please note that in the vast majority of golfers I see, it's not just about the swing. Even the most avid of golfers spend more time off the course than they do on it. What you do off the course can have just as big an impact – or even more impact – than what you do on it. For many golfers, tweaking their golf swing isn't the answer. As we'll see in Part 4, tweaking your life off the course can prove productive.

CASE STUDY: Introducing a car cushion

Robert had cut his golf right back to the point where he was wondering whether it was worth it or not. He often felt tired in his lower back after eighteen holes, but by the time he had driven the thirty minutes home, he struggled to get out of the car. It took a few days for his back to settle down enough to consider playing again.

I thought the drive rather than the golf was the bigger part of Robert's problem. By following my recommendation to sit on a cushion in the car, he discovered his lower back was no worse on getting out of the car than it was immediately after his round. That cushion enabled him to get back to two to three rounds a week instead of just the one.

Summary

- You must reduce or modify your Aggravators and Triggers.

- Golf swings can exert up to eight times your body weight on the lower back.

- The classic swing exerts less load on the back than the X-Factor Swing.

- Shortening backswing or slowing down can reduce back pain.

- Off-course activities impact back pain significantly.

- Lifestyle adjustments, such as using a car cushion, can alleviate post-game discomfort.

5
Risks

This bridging chapter looks forward from the Relief phase to the Prevention phase. We'll get more deeply into this stuff and what to do about it in Part 4, but in the meantime, we'll work on massively upgrading your understanding. Without that understanding, I'm willing to bet you won't stick with the programme, and that would be a shame. You'd have wasted the time you've spent reading up to this point, and the money you've invested in this book.

Once you have the understanding, you will be well equipped to move into Prevention mode, but before we do that, we need to look at the Risks. What are the risk factors for LBP (remember that most sciatica is as a result of a lower back problem)?

Primary and secondary risk factors

A slight technical point here – it's important that you understand this. Primary risk factors increase the risk of you having your first-ever episode of LBP. Secondary risk factors increase the risk of you becoming a persistent sufferer. The table below lists possible primary and secondary factors for LBP.

Primary and secondary risk factors for LBP

Primary risk factors	Secondary risk factors
Loading – peak, cumulative and sustained	Previous back pain
Trauma	Lower level of back muscle endurance
Whole body vibration	Low mood – anxiety/ depression
Lower level of back muscle endurance	Stress
Work-related 'stress'	Obesity
Smoking	Passive coping/ catastrophising
Age – over 40	
Lower levels of physical fitness and activity	

Note the appearance of 'passive coping/catastrophising' in the secondary risk factors, not the primary list – the reasons for this will become clear in Part 3. 'Whole body vibration' refers to driving or using heavy machinery – tractors, diggers, excavators, jackhammers. Lower levels of physical activity and of back muscle endurance later tie in with the first Rule of Rehabilitation (see Chapter 9).

The three types of loading

There are three types of loading, which are as follows:

1. **Peak load** is internal (you lift something heavy) or external (you get kicked in the back).

2. **Cumulative load** is a lighter load that you do repeatedly, eg a golf swing (although it could be argued this is internal peak loading, given the large forces involved in a full swing).

3. **Sustained load** is staying in one position for a prolonged period of time, eg sitting, driving or standing.

TOP TIP

If golf (cumulative loading) is an issue for you, remember you don't have to pull your driver out on every par 4 and 5. A full swing with a driver creates much more force (load) on your lower back than a cheeky little four iron off the tee.

Loading will fatigue the tissues at different rates. Your muscles will fatigue, your ligaments may fatigue, even the fibres of your discs will fatigue. You need to give them recovery time so that they don't fatigue to the point of pain or ultimately to the point of failure.

By understanding the physiology of different tissues (muscles, ligaments, tendons, bones, discs) we can optimise their recovery and help to make them stronger.

CASE STUDY: Loading problems

Joanna had been declining invitations to golf for a few years. A brief spell as a pro early in life had been followed by decades in the hospitality industry. Somewhere along the way, LBP had become an issue for her. It normally wasn't too bad at the end of the round, but after sitting for an hour in the clubhouse, she usually felt a lot worse.

It was the combination of golf and sitting that was the problem, not just the swing. This was cumulative and sustained loading at work.

Loading is *the* key risk for the initiation of most first-time LBP events; it's just not always that obvious. Most people don't develop LBP or sciatica purely because of stress, or smoking, or just because they're over 40. Remember that these are Risks; that is not the same as being a cause. You overload your lower back in one or a combination of the above ways (peak, cumulative or sustained), which triggers your pain, and that's your first episode. You can see that the secondary risks include more psychological and social factors, which we'll get into in Part 3.

If you want to reduce the risk of recurrence, ie you want to move as far back from the edge of the Cliff of Pain (see Chapter 2) as possible, you are going to have to address your Risks. What should you do? Reduce or modify them in some way so that they don't have as big a role to play in your future life. We'll learn how to do that in Part 4.

I'll say it again, Relievers are not enough. To move back from the edge, you must reduce or modify your Risks. Of course, it's easier said than done. If you'd like support in building your own plan for relief and prevention of your LBP or sciatica, come to one of our free workshops. Go to https://golf.painfreeandconfident.com/book-reader or scan the QR code below:

Pessimism can lead to persistent pain

Pessimistic golfers are less likely to win. It's a fact. Even when they do win, they don't enjoy the win as much – often putting it down to luck. The same is true with pain. As far as pain is concerned, a bad attitude is worse than a bad injury. The research is clear on this. Those who believe they are destined to a life of suffering are more likely to have exactly that. If you are known to be a worrier, with higher-than-average levels of anxiety, this could be one of your biggest barriers to recovery.

One reason is that you're less likely to do what needs to be done to recover. If you believe that it's beyond your ability to influence the outcome (this is known as a low level of self-efficacy), that will probably prove to be the case. The other reason is that you are literally heightening your levels of pain by focusing negatively on them. Researchers have found that one mechanism that can increase – and maintain – pain is how much you think about it.

Mentally focusing on something causes a release of a specific neurochemical called acetylcholine into the part of the brain that is processing the sensations. This reinforces the connections made between nerve cells (neurons). The more you focus on pain, the more you reinforce its presence (Chapman, Tuckett and Song, 2008). Put simply, the more you think about your pain, the more pain you will feel now and the more you're likely to feel in the future.

This is an important point: I am not saying that your pain is 'all in your head'. I know it started in your back or sciatic area, but the more pessimistic you are, the harder it will be to resolve your pain. Don't worry if that's you, we'll address it soon – please be patient;

we're nearly there. Remember it's important to fully understand where you've been going wrong; that way you're more likely to follow the plan when we finally come to it.

This can often be the elephant in the room, so I wanted to get it out into the open in these first chapters. You need to believe that there's a solution. If you don't, it's like tying one hand behind your back and still expecting to go round in par. You'll see later that this ties in exactly to one of the six Essential Practices.

The headline here is that the psychological and social factors (what you think and the relationships you have) much more strongly predict your likelihood of having long-term pain than what's happened in your back. This is not to shame you or annoy you. Don't shoot the messenger; I am merely reporting facts. Let's see how this situation develops by reviewing a widely accepted model.

Fear is the enemy

In 1983, a group of four researchers (Lethem, Slade, Troup and Bentley) first published what they called the 'Fear Avoidance Model'. It was specifically intended to explain why some LBP sufferers went on to become persistent sufferers and others didn't. See if it resonates with you.

Disuse/disability/depression ——————— Pain   Recovery

Avoidance of activity   Confrontation

Fear of pain   Pain experience   No fear

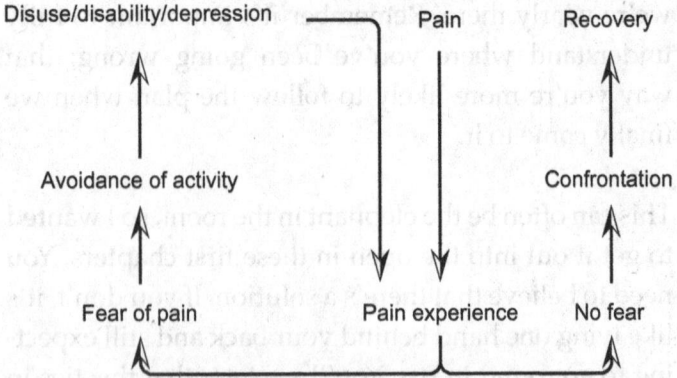

5.1 Lethem, Slade, Troup and Bentley's
Fear Avoidance Model, 1983, © Little T889, https://commons.
wikimedia.org/wiki/File:Fear-avoidance_model.jpg

As I will keep repeating, your thoughts and beliefs have a huge impact on the severity of your pain and suffering. What you think determines your behaviour, which in turn affects how you are likely to feel and what you are likely to do to bring about your recovery. This can cause a vicious circle, as shown above.

The more you fear your pain, the less you do, the weaker you become and the more likely your pain is to be triggered. Of course, many golfers – desperate to keep playing – will use painkillers to do so, relieving their pain and reducing their anxiety and disability as a result. This is rarely a workable long-term plan. For a variety of reasons, masking the pain with drugs to do more of what would otherwise be painful often leads to a long-term deterioration. It just delays the disability rather than avoiding it. Overuse of painkillers can lead to side effects such as stomach or kidney problems and even addiction (see Chapter 3).

Fear tends to lead to more disability, but what if your pain is worthy of fear? What if it's so damn sore that you would do anything to avoid it? Like using a ball pickup attachment on the end of your putter or even having to ask your mate to tee up your ball for you. That's a sad state of affairs, isn't it? For most golfers, it's avoidable.

TRY IT YOURSELF

Create a positive mantra, eg 'My back is getting stronger', and recite it to yourself many times each day.

In the meantime, what if your pain keeps happening? You can't just talk yourself out of fear, can you? No.

We fear the unknown much more than we fear the known, don't we? If you knew why you were in pain and what you could do yourself to take control, that would lessen the suffering, wouldn't it? Certainly that's what the evidence indicates.

CASE STUDY: The power of reassurance

Margaret had suffered what she described as 'excruciating pain' in her lower back and down the back and outside of her right thigh and lower leg for six weeks before consulting me. Based in Florida, she had consulted a chiropractor and two doctors in the last four weeks and had a battery of tests, an armful of drugs and felt anxious all the time, on top of the terrible pain. She had the impression her doctor thought she was a surgical case, although the chiro didn't.

Running through her history, a movement screen and her test results with her, I was able to reassure her that if she followed the guidance I gave her, she would feel significant improvements within the next ten days. She emailed me the next day to say that she already felt much better for having spoken to me, and that her pain levels had dropped by 30%.

Was this because her tissues had suddenly healed by 30% or was she just less fearful and more hopeful? It's unlikely this 30% drop was due to a reduction in pain inputs in her lower back and sciatic area. Much more likely it was due to her nervous system calming down a little.

Can you have fear and hope at the same time? Yes – just as you can be scared and brave simultaneously. Hope without fear is much more positive, and – as I keep saying – what you think can play a big role in your pain and recovery.

In another interesting study (Shimo *et al.*, 2011), it was demonstrated that showing images of a man carrying a heavy suitcase with a stooped posture triggered pain in people who had previously suffered persistent LBP. These painful sensations were also reflected in the functional MRIs of their brains, which showed that the low back sensory processing and emotional processing centres 'lit up' when these sufferers were shown the images of the crouching, suitcase-carrying man.

It seems that even being exposed to images of others performing 'risky' manoeuvres can be enough to increase pain; therefore, it may be necessary to inoculate yourself against 'scary'-looking images and activities. The field of LBP research is enormous. Due to it being so common, LBP costs society a huge amount. We've covered a fair bit of the science already, but we'll continue dipping in and out of it as you progress from painful and fragile to pain-free and confident.

Summary

- There are three types of loading – peak, cumulative and sustained – which can all contribute to Risk.

- There are numerous known Risks for the initial onset of pain (primary risk factors).

- There are other Risks for progressing to persistent pain (secondary risk factors).

- To make a sustainable recovery, you have to reduce your risk factors.

- One of the greatest Risks for long-term pain is fear – this must be overcome.

PART THREE
UNDERSTANDING

6
The Pain Equation

In this chapter, we will solve the puzzle of pain. Why do you hurt as much as you do? Why does pain vary? Why is it sometimes predictable and at other times totally unpredictable? How does pain work?

This stage is fairly science-heavy, but if you hated science at school, don't worry. I'm going to unpack the intricacies of pain by telling you a story involving a cyclist and a wasp. Sounds random, doesn't it? You can only truly master your pain by understanding it. When you read this story, you'll begin to move from student to master. Let's dive in, shall we?

The cyclist and the wasp

The cyclist in this story is me. The wasp plays a minor role. Let's begin.

In 2019, I was cycling to work early one summer's morning along idyllic, quiet country roads. The sun was climbing in the sky to my right and the birds were in full song in the trees around me. This is one of the best times of my working day. Especially when it's sunny, rather than windy and wet. Life felt good.

Suddenly, my thoughts were interrupted by a sharp jab of pain halfway up the front of my right thigh. I looked down to see a wasp sitting on my cycle shorts. I'd been stung. Brushing the wasp off, I had an opportunity to observe my own experience of pain. I still had forty minutes of cycling ahead of me, so I had plenty of time. Here is a collection of some of my thoughts as I cycled on towards work.

'Ow, that's sore. Never mind, I've been stung before. It's not a big deal.' (Pain level 2)

'Watch out, you crazy badger! Nearly ran you over there.' (Pain level 0)

'How's my thigh? It's still sore. I wonder if it's swelling. Yep, swelling already.' (Pain level 3)

'Busy junction coming up. Better pay attention to the traffic. He's coming slowly. I can get out in front of him. I need some serious effort to get up this hill.' (Pain level 0)

'The road's quieter now. Wonder how my thigh's doing? Still sore, though not too bad. No worse than ten minutes ago. I wonder if I'll have an anaphylactic shock response? I've never had one before due to a wasp sting but my lips and tongue swelled up a few years ago when I ate that hazelnut. It's a good thing I'm not far from the hospital.' (Pain level 5)

'Busy traffic. That guy cut me up on purpose. What an ****.' (Pain level 0)

My pain levels had varied between 0 and 5 on a scale of 0–10, averaging 2–3. As soon as I got into work, I made notes on my observations. Thinking about my pain levels, and what caused them to vary, led to the Pain Equation.

The Pain Equation solved

$$P = (N - MWP) + (NT - PT) + ATBP + PVOP$$

This is the Pain Equation. Don't be put off if you don't like maths – there's no need to be good at numbers to understand this equation. Let's break it down.

P represents the level of pain you experience at any given moment. Simple.

N means nociception. When something bad happens to your body, little nerve-endings called 'nociceptors' detect noxious events such as physical trauma, extremes of temperature or chemical changes (like inflammation). The nociceptors in the area fire off and send an electrical impulse to the next neuron (nerve cell), which starts in the spinal cord and runs up towards the brain. Nociception is a variable in the equation for pain: the more damage or inflammation, the more nociceptive input you're likely to have.

The wasp released a toxin into my thigh. This caused nociceptors to fire and inflammation to build up, triggering more nociceptive activity. Although the swelling and inflammation will have increased during my cycle and then remained fairly constant over the next two days, the pain didn't – it varied a lot, both during my cycle and over the next two days. It was rarely the same from one minute to the next. That's because of the other variables.

MWP means movement without pain. Why do you rub something that hurts? Why do you jump around when you hit your thumb with a hammer or stub your toe? Because the more movement you can do that doesn't cause pain, the less pain you're likely to feel. Ronald Melzack and Patrick Wall (1965) first described this as the Gate Control Theory.

When you move or press on part of your body, you stimulate sensory neurons called mechanoreceptors. They detect movement and pressure within tissues, and when they fire they block nociceptor messages. The next neurons in the pain pathways in your spinal cord and brain don't fire. Brilliant, isn't it? TENS (see Chapter 3), often used by women in labour, uses this system to reduce pain. By stimulating your mechanoreceptors, the TENS blocks the nociceptive input.

In addition to this mechanism, if you move around enough, your brain releases chemicals that suppress your pain system (this is a different mechanism). You typically need to exercise for longer to trigger the release of these chemicals. (There's a debate about whether endorphins or endocannabinoids are responsible for this.) Movement can reduce the nociceptive input into the spinal cord via the gate control. It can suppress it via these naturally occurring chemicals coming down from the brain. When I was cycling hard, I didn't feel any pain; this was the gate control at work (in addition to another mechanism below).

NT means negative thoughts (eg stress). If you are prone to depression, anxiety or feeling stressed, you're likely to experience more pain. Psychological and social (psychosocial) factors are stronger predictors of long-term pain. This is how. The pain pathways pass through the parts of your brain responsible for emotions and motivation. Your most powerful motivating emotion is fear. Worrying is an expression of fear. The more worry or fear you have, the more active this system is, and that augments your pain-pathway activity. Your pain system and emotional centres share neurons, so if fear is 'firing', pain is more likely to fire too.

I like to describe stress as fear; for example, fear you won't get paid this month, fear you'll lose your job and you won't be able to pay your mortgage, or fear you might get sick or perform badly at work. You may not be facing those fears consciously, but if you look inside yourself, they may well be there. When I was stressed, I felt more pain. It was no coincidence. When I thought about the possibility of anaphylaxis, my pain levels were at their highest.

The other reason persistent pain is worse in worriers is that the sensory processing of pain moves backwards in our brains the longer we have it. Where does it move to when it moves backwards? To the older parts of the brain that process emotions – our motivational centres. Perhaps this leaves the more recently evolved frontal parts of the brain to deal with more important matters.

PT means positive thoughts. Fortunately, a positive outlook can reduce pain. Your brain releases chemicals when you're enjoying yourself or connecting with other people in a positive way and these chemicals reduce your pain.

If you're feeling pain, do something you enjoy. Spend time with people you find uplifting, especially if you can move at the same time. Team sports, and dancing with a partner you like reduces pain levels dramatically, combining MWP and PT. When I remembered that I haven't had anaphylaxis previously and I'm generally lucky, my pain decreased immediately. When I revelled in the joy of cycling on a sunny summer's morning, I had no pain.

ATBP means attention to body part. The more you think about it, the more it will hurt. Attention to pain has a greater impact than anxiety. When you're busily engaged in something else, you feel less pain. Conversely, the more you focus on your pain, the worse it feels. Many people feel worse pain at night when there are no distractions. Whenever my attention drifted back to my thigh, the pain increased.

PVOP means previous volume of pain. I'm using 'volume' to mean two things: the amount of pain (cumulative over time) and its loudness (severity). The more pain you've experienced in the past, the more likely you are to feel pain – whether in the same body part or elsewhere. For example, migraine sufferers get more LBP and LBP sufferers get more migraines. Migraine sufferers get more repetitive strain injuries, and so on. The more severe your pain has been in the past, the more likely it is to recur. If you've had severe LBP, you're more likely to have another bout when compared with someone who's only had mild LBP.

This is due to central sensitisation – when your central nervous system (your brain and spinal cord) becomes sensitive. This is an effect of neuroplasticity. It's how nociplastic pain comes about.

Your nervous system's capacity to adapt is essential to learning. When neurons fire, they make firmer connections with one another and those connections become more sensitive. If you want to learn anything (like a new language), neuroplasticity is essential. Neuroplasticity is your friend – except when it comes to pain. Due to neuroplasticity, the more nociception you experience, the more likely you are to learn pain.

I hadn't been stung in the thigh before and my previous experience of wasp stings was that they're benign and don't cause many problems.

My pain is much worse

You might think, 'You only had a little wasp sting. My LBP is severe and debilitating. It's agony.'

You're right. Your LBP and level of nociceptive input is different to mine, but regardless of the amount of damage, the equation still applies.

In extreme cases, there can be a huge amount of nociceptive input, but they frequently don't result in any pain (at least at first). Shark attack victims frequently state they felt something 'hit' them under the water, but they didn't experience pain at the time, even when losing a limb. Perhaps this is partly because they didn't know they had been bitten, as it all happened underwater without them knowing there was a shark in the vicinity. This certainly causes a lot of nociceptive input but no pain, until they come out of the water and see the injury. At the other end of the spectrum, you can have severe pain with little or no nociceptive input.

We will now bring the Pain Equation alive with examples and help you apply it to your own challenges.

Pain and threat

This is the story – reported in the *British Medical Journal* (1995) – of a twenty-nine-year-old builder who jumped down onto an upturned nail. The nail passed straight through his boot, with the point appearing behind the steel toe-capped area, around the base of his big toe. On arrival at the accident and emergency department – in great pain and upset – he was sedated with fentanyl midazolam and the nail was then removed.

All along, there was a puzzling absence of blood; perhaps his boot was holding it all. Now all was revealed. As the boot was cut off, the medical team discovered that the nail had passed *between* his toes, not even grazing his skin, yet he was in severe pain. Why? Because his brain told him that a nail had gone through his foot, and onlookers were suitably concerned (psychosocial), therefore the brain generated all of his pain. No nociceptive input or damage at all but lots and lots of pain.

Most people focus on what they imagine is the cause of their pain: 'tissue damage', but that's only the cause of your nociception. You expect the pain to have an entirely physical cause. It doesn't. I often say, 'No brain, no pain.' Your brain has the final say and determines how much pain you experience at any given time.

Look at the variables in the equation:

$$\text{Pain} = (N - MWP) + (NT - PT) + (ATBP) + (PVOP)$$

Most of them have nothing to do with 'tissue damage' – only nociception does – but NT, ATBP and PVOP have a lot to do with threat. Leading pain researchers agree that the amount of tissue damage is a poor predictor of the amount of pain you feel. Remember the shark attack victims? If you don't know you've been bitten, it doesn't hurt as much. Shark-bite victims who see the fin approaching them before they're bitten probably experience much more pain – just my guess. As for the poor embarrassed builder with the nail through his boot – his brain told him he had a nail in his foot. That's a strong threat, so it hurt – a lot.

Threat has a huge impact in determining how much pain you feel. Leading pain researchers have concluded that if you feel threatened by your pain, then your pain levels will be higher (Lorimer Moseley and Butler, 2015). If your pain threatens your ability to golf (and golf is important to you) then your pain is likely to be worse than if golf didn't matter to you.

The three types of pain

Pain scientists have recently proposed three types of pain. Let's deal with each of these in relation to the Pain Equation.

1. **Nociceptive pain.** This is pain that is caused by peripheral input, ie the firing of the nociceptors. Some people would call this straightforward pain. Arguably, most of my wasp-sting pain was nociceptive.

2. **Nociplastic pain.** This is pain that is caused by the central nervous system (and sometimes the peripheral nervous system) having been sensitised. It is the total of the other variables in the Pain Equation. The builder with the nail through his boot had nociplastic pain, with nothing coming from the nociceptors; it was all generated by his central nervous system.

3. **Neuropathic pain.** This is pain that is due to actual irritation of peripheral nerves. If you

have direct pressure on one of your lumbar spinal nerve roots this can cause a type of sciatica that is neuropathic (the most common cause being disc problems). Diabetes can cause damage to peripheral nerves, and this causes a diabetic neuropathy. Neuropathic pain isn't generally benefited by most painkillers. Other classes of drugs, such as amitriptyline and gabapentin (see Chapter 3), are often used for neuropathic pain.

As an example, if you have a disc prolapse affecting a spinal nerve and you've been in pain for even a few weeks, you will have nociceptive pain due to local inflammation triggering the nociceptors and neuropathic pain due to irritation of the spinal nerve. There's a good chance that your peripheral and central nerves will have been sensitised and you'll have some nociplastic pain too.

Duration of pain

While we're looking at pain terms, when most people say 'the pain is really acute' or 'it's chronic', they generally mean it's severe. In the worlds of pain science and clinical practice, acute and chronic have nothing to do with severity; they simply refer to duration. There is a bit of variation from country to country and between one organisation and another.

The framework we will use for duration of pain is:

- **Acute:** Lasting less than six weeks.
- **Subacute:** Lasting six to twelve weeks.
- **Chronic:** Lasting more than twelve weeks.

Negative thinking and pain

Don't forget that 'NT' in the Pain Equation refers to all negative thinking (stress), not just the thinking related to your back. What impact do you think all those various scary-sounding diagnoses have had on your pain over the years? You'll see why clinicians with a deep understanding of pain avoid these diagnoses if they can and only refer for MRIs and X-rays when absolutely necessary.

TRY IT YOURSELF

Try counting how often you think negatively about your lower back in a day. Do you refer to your back as 'weak', 'bad' or 'a problem'? All of those thoughts will reinforce your pain. Even describing yourself as a 'sufferer' may reinforce these pain pathways in your brain.

If you are to stop being a sufferer, you need to believe that it is possible to stop suffering and to change your identity from that of 'sufferer'. It

---

would be OK to say that you are someone who experiences pain, but 'sufferer' suggests a passive role. By following Part 4, you are not going to be passive in your experience of pain.

CASE STUDY: Anxious putting

Wilma was a sixty-two-year-old golfer who had to adopt a broomstick putter because stooping over her conventional putter caused her too much LBP. She admitted that she had always been an anxious putter. By working on her putting anxiety, her physical pain resolved too.

Pain is complex. It's not just due to what happens in your back, it's a summation of everything that's ever happened to you and what you think about it, consciously and unconsciously.

TRY IT YOURSELF

Armed with the Pain Equation, ask yourself: 'Why am I still in pain?' Remember that the body has the capacity to heal and recover from many serious injuries.

Mechanical labels for LBP

When I qualified as an osteopath, we viewed pain in the muscular and skeletal system as generally due to mechanical derangements. Explanations you might have been given for your pain could include some of the below:

- Twisted/tilted pelvis
- One leg longer than the other
- Muscle imbalances
- Subluxation
- Scoliosis
- Twisted spine
- Short or tight hamstrings
- Short or tight hip flexors
- Weak glutes
- Sway back
- Lordosis
- Kyphosis

These expressions and more are bandied around as explanations for pain. I did it myself for many years. We didn't know any better, but that's no excuse now. The evidence is clear: misalignments are not the cause. They may be associated with pain – it's quite common to find people with persistent LBP who have one or more from this list – but that doesn't mean these mechanical factors are the cause; they could just be coincidence or the consequence.

As tempting as these labels are for explaining pain, they are an oversimplification because pain is an interplay of many factors – the variables laid out in the Pain Equation. Admittedly, there are other subtleties; I'm not saying the Pain Equation is the only way to view pain but it has served me and thousands of others well. You can stick to your mechanical view of pain if you like, but it's the equivalent of being a flat-earther; pain science has moved on. I know something went wrong in your back and that was the original problem, but if you've had pain for years then it will no longer be purely nociceptive – it'll be nociplastic too. I guarantee it.

TRY IT YOURSELF

List all the diagnoses and explanations you've been given for your pain. Next time you get another one, ask the clinician, 'How exactly does that cause my pain? Is it possible to have this situation without pain?'

When a clinician or fitness professional asserts that a person's LBP is due to twisted pelvis/leg length difference/twisted spine/subluxation (or any from the above list), I always delight in asking them, 'How exactly does that cause pain?' Given that I'm asking someone who professes to know about these things, I am specifically wanting an answer that demonstrates their understanding of the neurophysiological processes. I've never had a satisfactory answer, when these mechanical 'diagnoses' are given. That is because many clinicians and the vast majority of fitness professionals do not understand how pain works. You do.

TOP TIP

If you haven't got your head round this, then please re-read this part of the book. Golfers who understand their pain are much more likely to overcome it.

Summary

- The Pain Equation gives you a framework for understanding how pain works:

$$P = (N - MWP) + (NT - PT) + ATBP + PVOP$$

  where N= nociception, MWP = movement without pain, NT = negative thoughts, PT = positive thoughts, ATBP = attention to body part and PVOP = previous volume of pain.

- Understanding can give you confidence, which enables you to overcome your fear. You need to understand your pain if you're to overcome your fear and regain any confidence in your back.

- Pain isn't just due to damaged tissues; it is complex. You can have damage without pain, and you can have pain without damage.

7

Further Understanding

This chapter gives a little more insight on important points for you to understand, debunking some myths along the way.

MRIs and other test results

If you're looking for certainty from an X-ray or MRI, you're in danger of being disappointed. It's totally normal to find 'abnormalities' in people who have no pain; in fact, 'abnormalities' are actually normal as you age. If you think your spine – or any part of your body – stays the same as you age, you are wrong. Look at your skin, your hair, your eyesight, your hearing – everything changes as we age. Disc bulges, prolapses and herniations are part of ageing (see the table below).

Age-specific prevalence estimates of degenerative lumbar spine imaging findings in asymptomatic patients (Brinjikji et al., 2015)

Age	Disc degeneration (%)	Disc height loss (%)	Disc bulge (%)	Disc protrusion (%)	Facet degeneration (%)	Spondylolisthesis (%)
20	37	24	30	29	4	3
30	52	34	40	31	9	5
40	68	45	50	33	18	8
50	80	56	60	36	32	14
60	88	67	69	38	50	23
70	93	76	77	40	69	35
80	96	84	84	43	83	50

As an example, in fifty year olds with no LBP or sciatica, the incidence of lumbar disc bulge is 60% and the incidence of degenerative changes is 80%. Remember that these numbers refer to the 'asymptomatic' population, ie people without any pain or other symptoms. There are lots of people wandering around with wear and tear and disc problems who have no pain at all. Just because your lower back is sore and there is wear and tear there does not mean that they are related.

MRI and CT scans can be helpful in confirming the likely cause of symptoms. They sometimes also show things we didn't expect but need to know (eg tumours, rarely). These investigations have been massively overused – especially in more affluent nations, such as the USA. Expensive investigations like these should never replace good clinical sense. They can be used to complement but should never replace a good assessment process (see Chapter 9).

Medicine is big business. There's a lot of money made from these investigations, and yes – for the record – I do think a lot of this is a poor use of hard-earned money/insurance premiums/tax.

Diagnoses doing harm

Remember that just by receiving a scary-sounding diagnosis, you are likely to suffer for longer than someone given a more benign explanation. Your diagnosis really can influence your long-term prospects, irrespective of what's actually wrong with your back. Having MRIs and other investigations can lead to more scary-sounding diagnoses.

The biopsychosocial model

A New York psychiatrist, Dr George Engel (1977) was the first to coin the term 'the biopsychosocial model'. It has been slow to catch on, but it is now certainly accepted universally as the gold standard by the pain science community and by the medical community specialising in pain. The biopsychosocial model explains illness and health as an interplay between three different realms:

1. Biological (what's happening in your lower back)

2. Psychological (your brain/mind)

3. Socio-environmental (your relationships and what's happening around you)

I'm pretty sure it was one of the many models introduced to me as an osteopathic student in the late 1980s. I'm equally sure that it was not put forward as the preferred model. It wasn't until I was studying for a Master's degree in The Clinical Management of Pain twenty years later that I read this was the gold standard and that it had been for three decades.

What I also rediscovered when studying for that degree was something many manual therapists conveniently forget: that the factors that predispose someone most strongly to developing long-term pain are psychosocial rather than biological. Remember the Fear Avoidance Model from Chapter 5? On top of that, people of an anxious or depressive nature have more trouble recovering from pain than those of a happier disposition. For persistent LBP sufferers, this is a more important factor than any actual damage in their backs. I am not saying it's all in your head – your back is definitely where the problem lies, but it's important to cover all the evidence so that we can build a plan for your long-term recovery. It's no use ignoring the science simply because it's unpalatable.

What determines the amount of pain we experience and how we recover from that pain is an interplay between biological, psychological and socio-environmental factors. This was fully laid out in the Pain Equation. If you struggle with the idea of body and mind being wholly integrated, how do you explain blushing – a physical manifestation of an emotion? Or the nail-in-the-boot guy? Also, what about phantom limb pain? Around 85% of amputees develop pain in a limb that no longer exists, where there is no nociception.

What goes wrong with backs?

In this part of the book, we've been pulling together the science behind pain. Let's get into the biological now and answer a few important questions:

- What has actually happened in your back?
- What is sciatica?
- How can you recover?

Nociceptive input and healing

We should work out whether you might still have nociceptive input going on and what to do about it.

TOP TIP

Remember that your back can recover from all sorts of injuries and weaknesses. Regardless of the damage to your back, there are plenty of reasons to be hopeful.

I am always more concerned by a long duration of symptoms than I am by the extent of damage. That's because of nociplastic pain. When your nervous system has learnt pain, it usually takes longer to unlearn it than it takes the tissues to heal from damage. The only diagnoses I'm going to dig into here are those involving discs and nerves, because recovering from all the other muscular and skeletal problems is more straightforward. Please take your time and read the next paragraph with all your attention.

Remember Doc Randall said, 'Many of your patients will get better, despite what you do to them'? That's because your body has the capacity to heal itself; just follow the Rules of Rehabilitation and it will heal.

There are thousands of systems operating in your body attempting to return you to optimal function – this is homeostasis, which is common across all living organisms, except viruses. Inflammation is one of those systems; it isn't a bad thing, it helps to fight infection and repair damaged tissues. In most cases of persistent pain, we have been messing up nature's attempts to heal us and return us to health. One assumption that I've made is that you have sufficient nutrition to heal.

If that important paragraph annoys you, I'm truly sorry. It's not your fault if you've been doing the wrong things. You've been following bad advice, based on a poor understanding of pain and rehabilitation, but that is all changing for you now. Whether you have a pulled muscle, a strained ligament, an inflamed tendon or even a bone fracture, if you do the right things – and avoid the wrong things – you can recover. In Chapter 9, I'll be providing you with a Functional Assessment, which is much more useful to you than a diagnosis.

Desperate discs and nipped nerves

There are lots of good images on the internet of intervertebral discs. One common comparison is that a lumbar disc is like a jam doughnut. In a disc, the doughy outer bit is tough and fibrous – it's called the annulus fibrosus. The jam in the middle is the nucleus pulposus, which is softer and gelatinous. Of course, the disc changes as we age, drying out a bit and flattening. This is what we see in X-rays and

MRIs of older spines (spines whose owners have no pain, remember).

Spinal nerves originate in the spinal cord and exit from the spine. In the lumbar spine, the nerves exit below their respective vertebrae. The L1 Nerve Root (L1NR) exists between L1 and L2 vertebrae, the L2NR exists between L2 and L3 vertebrae and so on. As we go down, we get to the sacral nerves. S1 exits between S1 and S2, which in adults are fused together. All five sacral vertebrae fuse together to form the sacrum in your teenage years.

Branches from the L4, L5, S1, S2 and S3 spinal nerves join together deep in the pelvis to form the sciatic nerve. I often describe the sciatic nerve as like the Amazon River – it's the biggest, longest nerve in your body and has a number of tributaries (L4–S3 spinal nerves).

Sciatica

Sciatica is pain and/or pins and needles and numbness in the distribution of your sciatic nerve. That's a big area. Pain caused by sciatica can include the buttocks, the back and outside of the thighs, the whole lower leg (except a strip down the front inner area to the inside ankle bone) and the whole of the foot. The pain can vary from an ache to a lightning pain shooting down the length of the nerve. Pins and needles may appear anywhere but are more common below the knee. The same is true of numbness. Some clinicians – like me – divide sciatica into two types.

1. **Nerve-irritation (compression) sciatica** – If your sciatic nerve or one of its tributaries is irritated or compressed, the pain (and any pins and needles) tends to be worse below the knee. Common causes of direct irritation or compression are disc bulges and degenerative changes. Rarely, it can be due to more serious medical pathology.

2. **Non-nerve-irritation (compression) sciatica** – This is referred pain, meaning that you feel the pain in the distribution of your sciatic nerve but it's not due to direct irritation or compression. It's because the tissue that the nociception is originating from has its nerve supply from one of the tributaries of the sciatic nerve. A bit like crossed-wires, the brain is perceiving the pain as coming from somewhere that it isn't coming from. That other site has the same nerve supply as the source of the pain. In non-nerve-irritation sciatica, the sciatic pain is usually worse above the knee.

A useful (though not foolproof) guide: if your sciatic pain is worse below the knee, it's usually nerve-irritation sciatica. If it's worse above the knee, it's usually non-nerve-irritation sciatica. Pins and needles below the knee also make it more likely that you have nerve-irritation sciatica.

There are a number of tests a good clinician would carry out to differentiate between these, including testing your muscle power, your reflexes and your sensation. They may also conduct a straight leg raise test. I am not going to unpack those tests here as we're not providing diagnosis services through a book.

Nipped nerve

When a nerve has been compressed or irritated directly, I call it a nipped nerve. When this happens, it can take the nerve many weeks to recover from this trauma. The pain of a nipped or compressed nerve is what was referred to earlier as neuropathic pain, ie coming from the nerve itself.

Even once the nipping has stopped, the nerve is still likely to be painful for quite a while afterwards. In these cases, pain isn't a good indicator of whether the problem is healing or not. You can be doing all the right things, but the pain is still there for a few weeks, even months.

When you have a nipped nerve, I'll always advise you that if you follow the plan, you can still improve. Be patient – it usually takes longer to see the plan paying off. Unlike most other problems, nipped nerves are slow to heal.

Disc bulges, herniations and prolapses

Intervertebral discs can go wrong. One way of looking at disc problems is to separate them into three categories:

1. **Degenerative discs** – Your discs wear as you get older but – as discussed earlier – you can have very worn discs and no pain. If your degenerative discs are contributing to your pain, you can expect this whole thing to take longer to improve than if you didn't have those degenerative changes. As the discs thin, the vertebrae get closer together. There are frequently also changes in the bones themselves. They often broaden out and develop bony spurs – bits of bone that grow out at the margins. This can result in less space for the nerve, increasing the chances of a nipped nerve. This type of change in discs and bones is often referred to as spondylosis, or spondylotic change. If there's inflammation too, the term is spondylitis.

2. **Discrete disc problems** – As described above, the annulus is the tough fibrous outer ring of a disc. It can tear – a simple tear of the disc is called an annular strain. It results in inflammation and must heal by the formation of new annular material to bind it all back together again. This is like scar tissue forming in your skin after a cut. The second level of disc injury is when enough of the fibres tear that the disc bulges. The nucleus pulposus is still contained within the outer rings of the disc but the disc has changed shape; it is now bulging. This bulge may displace the spinal nerve as it exits behind the disc.

3. **Disc prolapse** – This happens when enough of the fibres tear that some of the nucleus pulposus leaks out through the tear. Depending on how much space there is for this nuclear material, it may or may not compress the exiting spinal nerve. If it does, you're highly likely to have neuropathic pain as well as nociceptive pain, and likely will develop nociplastic pain too. Don't worry, all of these can be resolved by following a good rehab plan.

Disc bulges often swell when you are lying down. Consequently, many people feel worse at night and first thing in the morning. Inflammation of the disc is also likely to build up overnight, making the pain worse when you wake up. The key thing with desperate discs and nipped nerves is that you are trying to rehab two different tissues – the disc and the nerve. Sometimes the two benefit from different movements. The Rules of Rehabilitation always apply.

Tears and bulges in our discs are normal as we age. It's the speed that these events happen at – and the resulting inflammation – that determines how much nociception we experience. What we're always looking for is how much nipping of the nerve is happening.

CASE STUDY: Large disc prolapse

Jennifer has had four lumbar disc surgeries. After her third, the surgeon said it was a large disc prolapse and that Jennifer had large nerves and small spaces between the bones. Therefore, there was a lot of pressure on the L5 spinal nerve.

Most of us will be luckier than Jennifer – smaller prolapse, smaller nerves and lots of space is a recipe for much less neuropathic pain.

Special considerations when rehabbing discs

As mentioned in Chapter 4, discs do not have a direct blood supply so they are slow to heal. They also don't have a direct nerve supply so you often don't know when you are aggravating them.

In the short term, stick to activities that will not stretch the original tear; that way you will allow the scar tissue to form fully. For most of us, the tear is at the back of the disc, near the nerve. In the short term, that means not bending forwards or twisting and definitely not combining the two.

TRY IT YOURSELF

Most people bend forwards in their lower backs when they sit. Don't do that. Maintain the arch in the small of your back, to allow the disc time to heal.

If you're struggling to recover from a lumbar disc problem and you're doing forward-bending stretches, stop them. If you are bending forwards to tie shoelaces, get on socks or load the dishwasher, stop that too.

I call these actions 'picking the scab before it's ready to fall off' – it will bleed and re-scab. Give the disc time to heal. There's more on this in the free online Rapid Relief Plan (see Chapter 3 for QR code).

TOP TIP

If you definitely have a disc problem which is nipping a nerve, ask yourself if you're giving each of those tissues the optimum conditions for healing. Make sure you aren't 'picking the scab too early'.

Summary

- MRIs and X-rays can throw up red herrings.
- Diagnoses can do harm, prolonging recovery time.
- Your back can recover physically from many injuries if you follow the right plan.
- There are two types of sciatica.
- Discs do not have a direct blood supply, meaning they are slow to heal.
- Discs do not have a direct nerve supply, so you may not know you are injuring one.
- Rehabilitating discs and nerves is slower and more complicated.
- Make sure you aren't 'picking the scab too early'.

8
My Own Journey With Back Pain And Sciatica

This chapter personalises everything you've learnt so far. I hope there are parts of my story that resonate with you. I include it to clarify how to apply the Cliff of Pain model (see Chapter 2).

My LBP and sciatica story

I first strained my lower back close to my nineteenth birthday, lifting heavy weights in the gym. I got better over a period of around two weeks. It got sore again, then it got better, then it got sore, then it spread into my left thigh and the outside of my lower leg. The timescales on this are a little vague (it's thirty-six years ago), but certainly all of this happened within the first year.

My pain was typically triggered by forward-bending movements, most of them totally innocuous like reaching forward to lift a glass off a low table or bending over to lock my bike to a railing (Triggers). When my back and leg were sore, they were clearly aggravated by sitting and also by bending forwards, eg I always struggled to get my socks on (Aggravators). The pain was always worse in the mornings (inflammation and the disc bulge swelling overnight). This went on episodically for years.

Massage and manipulation usually helped it to feel better (Relievers). I rarely used medication but did when I had severe, incapacitating flare-ups. On these occasions – which lasted a few days at the 9/10 pain level – I could barely move and was pretty distressed. I did quite a bit of stretching because it felt good at the time (and I was advised to by numerous clinicians). Later, I would learn that this probably slowed down my recovery.

My sciatica was fairly constant for a few years but became less of an issue when I started avoiding sitting as much as possible. My LBP also settled down a lot when I minimised sitting (avoiding/reducing Aggravators). It seems crazy to me now, but avoiding or minimising sitting was such a breakthrough for me. I used to sit down in lectures for as long as I could bear – ten to twenty minutes – then get up and pace around at the back. Simply by not sitting in the first place, I had far less pain. What I didn't know was that by sitting I was preventing the back of my disc from healing, and re-inflaming it, hence my lack of progress.

Once I stopped doing this (I'd already adapted forward bending), I was able to start to heal. I could start to rebuild the strength and robustness of my back (Preventers). Given how easily I had flare-ups when bending forwards, I suspect now that I had marked instability in my lower back, but no one was talking about it then so I didn't even know it was a thing. Once I had regained the cliff top and realised what my silent risk factors were, minimised those and started practising some Preventer exercises, I made real progress in getting back from the edge.

Other interesting points from my history

A few years into my persistent/recurrent LBP and sciatica, I noticed that stress became an Aggravator. On one occasion, it was a clear Trigger.

All had been well with my back for a year or so, and then my second son was diagnosed with a lifelong medical condition. I distinctly remember sitting in the haematology consultant's office, listening intently to the words that I felt were going to determine the course of his life. Like the Otago student's flat, my memories of that consultation are clear. I remember the room was messy; stacks of papers everywhere (this was twenty-five years ago). It was an old building too with a damp smell. The computer system took about five minutes to crank into gear – longer than it took the consultant to break the news. As I walked out of the consultant's office, I noticed my back was aching. Within an hour, it was 7/10 pain.

At the time I thought, 'On top of the stress of dealing with this, somehow I've also strained my back.' The pain was significant and exactly the same as previous episodes. It wasn't until my back pain settled down a few days later that it dawned on me I hadn't had my usual forward-bending or sitting trigger. The only possible Trigger I could think of was the stress. This is typical of nociplastic pain. Remember the Pain Equation (see Chapter 6) – negative thinking (aka stress) can certainly contribute to pain. In this case, it was the sole Trigger, which when combined with my previous volume of pain was enough to flare up my pain pathways. This is common in people with persistent or recurrent pain.

My final straw

When I was twenty-seven, I was changing my nephew's nappy, kneeling on the floor. It wasn't the first time, so it only took a few minutes. Of course, changing a six-month-old boy's nappy is a bit of a stressful wrestling match. When I stood up from that bending-forward position, my lower back was achy. By this time, I had had seven-plus years of on/off LBP and sciatica. My wife and I were due our first child in about three months. I knew there were a lot of forward bending, carrying and awkward positions coming my way.

This was the final straw. This was the moment when I made the commitment to do whatever was necessary to 'fix' my back, to build my back to be as strong as I could get it. Although I had already formulated the Cliff of Pain years earlier, this was the moment when I totally committed to get as far back from the edge as possible. This is the importance of having a framework: it gives you a map to plan for – what, up until now, has been an elusive, hope-fuelled, long-term solution. In the next part of the book, we are going to cover Prevention – getting right back from the edge.

Summary

- Sometimes Triggers are obvious, sometimes not.
- Aggravators need to be avoided to enable recovery.
- Relievers vary but only relieve.
- Addressing the Risks enabled me to get back from the edge.
- Strengthening my lower back helped (Preventer exercises).
- Sometimes you need a significant episode or future event to give you the motivation to stick to the plan.

PART FOUR
PREVENTION

9
Essential Practice 1: Measure

I n this chapter, we will focus on the first of the six Essential Practices: Measure. We delve into the value of measuring and what to measure – there are broadly two types of measuring and we'll cover both. We will also unveil the first Rule of Rehabilitation.

If you are skim-reading this book, or you've just jumped straight here because you can't be bothered with Part 3, I understand your thinking, but please go back and work through the book methodically or it's highly likely your pain will recur. Without a foundational understanding, your progress will be built on shaky ground.

If it matters, measure it

On the Cliff of Pain (see Chapter 2), the label 'Preventers' refers to the six Essential Practices. They may not all be essential to you achieving a long-term solution, but I have seen enough former sufferers of LBP practising one (usually three-plus) of these to know that they warrant your serious attention.

TOP TIP

If you want to get right back from the edge, practise as many of the six Essential Practices as you can. I don't know who first said it, but 'practice doesn't make perfect; it makes habits.'

You could say that a diagnosis is a type of measurement. From what I've unveiled in Chapter 7, you might feel that diagnosis seems to be futile, but there is definitely value in some diagnostic measuring. When you consult a clinician and give an update, they will often ask, 'How have you been?' This often triggers a long description of your latest flare-up, or tales of visiting your mother-in-law and how soft her mattress is. You have focused on one event, and – truth be told – the clinician doesn't really know whether you're improving or not, or why. We need a measure of your pain, because without one we don't really know whether you're progressing or not.

Pain is difficult to quantify, isn't it? That's what you'll often hear. I don't agree. Many clinicians use the Numeric Pain Rating Scale (NPRS) – a scale of 0 (no pain) to 10 (worst possible pain). It is purely a measure of severity. It says nothing about the quality of your pain, but it's a reasonable guide of progress within an individual. You can give an average NPRS over the last twenty-four hours, or you could give your worst NPRS in the last week, or both. This is what we do in clinical practice. We ask our patients: 'What has your average pain been over the last twenty-four hours?' and 'What has been your highest pain level over the last week?' Both on a 0–10 scale.

Whatever timescale you use; it is pointless to compare one person's pain rating with another's. Your pain is your pain and it's real to you. Whatever number you put on it, it is your number. The same is true for me and my pain.

Using the NPRS can be a useful snapshot of pain severity, and it can be tracked over time. This means we can measure your progress.

TRY IT YOURSELF

Take a minute and write down your average pain over the last twenty-four hours, and your highest pain over the last week.

The Backscore

Another measure – one I've found to be more valuable – is measuring the impact that pain has on your life. These measurements are generically referred to as disability measures. How much are you 'disabled' by your pain? This doesn't have to mean 'wheelchair-bound' disabled; it could simply mean that you can't get up and down the stairs easily, for example.

The measure I have used for twenty years is the Roland–Morris Disability Questionnaire, a clinically validated tool (Roland and Morris, 1983). There are others, but I like the simplicity of this one. Ten years ago, Professor Roland (now retired) gave me permission to use it (thank you very much, Prof Roland) in reverse – as a measure of ability. To call it 'The Backscore'. In the *Pain-Free & Confident* programmes, we use The Backscore as a measure of how able you are to go about everyday activities (like go up and down stairs).

You want your Backscore to be as close to 100 as possible. The idea is you mark all the statements as either true or false and at the end you get a score. Here are just three of the statements:

1. I get dressed more slowly than usual because of my back.

2. I only stand for short periods of time because of my back.

3. Because of my back, I try not to bend or kneel down.

When we take on a new client, we always get them to do their Backscore, and retest to demonstrate progress every few weeks.

You can get your own Backscore by visiting https://getbackscore.scoreapp.com or scanning the QR code:

If you've had pain for years (as many of our patients have), it's useful to track your Backscore. This gives a more objective measure of the impact your back is having on your life. Therefore, it's easier to track changes over time.

I was tempted to create a disability measure that included your pain's impact on your ability to golf, but it wouldn't be a validated measure if I did that and I'd prefer to use a validated measure than a half-baked one. To borrow from Peter F Drucker (*The Effective Executive*) in the world of business, 'What gets measured, gets improved.' I also love the title of John Doerr's book, *Measure What Matters*. Measuring pain isn't terribly effective in improving your long-term outcomes. If you want to measure what matters, measure your Backscore.

TRY IT YOURSELF

Record your own NPRS (0–10) and get your Backscore. Write them down or put them on a spreadsheet and track them over time.

Your Functional Assessment

Remember that thinking in purely mechanical terms (twisted pelvis, tilted spine, etc) isn't helpful. There's little point in measuring leg lengths, postural tilts or how tight your hamstrings or hip flexors are. MRIs are of questionable benefit, unless you're having to consider surgery, and X-rays are almost useless. It's vitally important to measure your progress – if you have a goal, you should be measuring your progress towards it using the NPRS and The Backscore.

You may also remember how many people are confused by multiple diagnoses. Some find them downright scary. Consequently, a diagnosis can do more harm than good; they certainly don't empower you. Is there a useful alternative to a diagnosis? A label that provides powerful insights and empowers you?

Yes, there is.

During my MSc in Pain Management, I proposed a labelling system that would inform clinicians and empower patients. I called it a 'Functional Assessment'. I am certainly not the only clinician to use an assessment based on function. This is not a novel concept. This particular Functional Assessment is my own combination of factors that I have used in my clinical practice for over ten years to label LBP and sciatica. Here's how it works.

Location

Where is your pain?

- Lower back and buttock area = Lumbago

- Back or outside of thigh; the back, outside and front of the lower leg; and the top and outside and sole of foot = Sciatica

(Front or inside of thigh, inside of lower leg and inside of ankle is not within the sciatic distribution, so if you have pain there, it's not sciatica.)

Duration

If you have LBP/buttock pain, how long have you had this episode of pain?

If you have pain in the sciatic distribution, how long have you had this episode of pain?

- Less than six weeks = Acute
- Six to twelve weeks = Subacute
- More than twelve weeks = Chronic

Recurrent

Which of the below is most accurate?

- I've had this one, and one previous episode of pain in the last year = Single Recurrent
- I've had more than two episodes of this pain in the last year = Multiple Recurrent

If you have only had this one episode of pain in the last year, you can leave this element out.

Directional preference/intolerance

If you have LBP, which of the below is most likely to make your LBP worse?

If you have sciatic distribution pain, which of the below is most likely to make this pain worse?

- Sitting or getting up from sitting or bending forwards = Flexion Intolerant

- Standing/walking or bending backwards = Extension Intolerant

- Both of the above equally = Flexion and Extension Intolerant

- Neither = Leave blank

Instability

Do you get a sharp pain in your lower back when you turn over in bed or change position?

- Yes = With Instability

- No = Leave blank

Here are some examples of Functional Assessments:

- LBP for four months, which is worse for sitting and it hurts turning over in bed: Chronic Flexion Intolerant Lumbago with Instability.

- Pain in sciatic distribution (no LBP) for the last three weeks, third episode this year, which is aggravated by standing and bending backwards: Acute Multiple Recurrent Extension Intolerant Sciatica.

- Six months of lower back and buttock pain, worse for bending forwards. Had previous episode within last twelve months, and two weeks of sciatic distribution pain, which is worse when standing: Chronic Single Recurrent Flexion Intolerant Lumbago and Acute Extension Intolerant Sciatica.

TRY IT YOURSELF

Record your own Functional Assessment, based on the framework above. It will be invaluable in guiding you in what to do and what not to do.

Note there may be different duration and intolerance labels for lumbago and sciatica, as in the last example.

You might be asking 'What is the value of each element of the Functional Assessment?' I'm glad you asked.

- **Location** – This makes it clear to everyone what we're dealing with, without freaking you out. Lumbago simply means LBP.

- **Duration** – The longer you've had a pain, usually the longer it takes to resolve it under the optimal circumstances.

- **Recurrent** – The more episodes you've had, the longer it tends to take to resolve under the optimal circumstances.

- **Directional preference/intolerance** – Coming back to the Aggravator issue, if it hurts to do something, you should reduce that activity. (Reducing is one of the six Essential Practices, see

Chapter 10.) If you are Flexion Intolerant, you need to reduce sitting and forward bending (at least during the Relief phase).

* **Instability** – If you have instability, there are particular exercises that are likely to improve matters for you. Stretching is almost certainly a no-no.

TOP TIP

Your intolerance is particularly important because it tells you which daily activities and movements you should be reducing in the short term. It also indicates which exercises are most likely to relieve your pain.

If you want to get better, it helps to measure progress. That takes us to a different type of measuring: tracking.

Tracking Aggravators, Triggers, Risks, Relievers and Preventers

The measure practice is not only about providing fixed labels, it's also about tracking. I encourage you to monitor your behaviour. It's well documented that simply tracking your behaviour leads to a change in behaviour. A good example is using a step tracker. As soon as people start tracking their steps, many people start trying to get more in, sometimes going to great lengths to hit higher targets. It's the same with calorie counting; just by counting, you tend to reduce.

You only have to look at your Cliff of Pain to find things you may wish to track, ie Aggravators, Triggers, Risks (or the behaviours associated with them), Relievers and Preventers. Equally, the Pain Equation (see Chapter 6) provides you with another list of things you may wish to track – movement without pain, mood, etc.

Aggravators and Triggers

Many people find it helpful to track their Aggravators and Triggers. Often, these are things we do habitually – like sitting. It helps to bring them to the top of the mind. Again, just tracking them often changes your frequency and duration of doing them.

Risks

This is a super-important part of the book. You've seen the table below in Chapter 5. Here it comes again. Get yourself a cup of your preferred beverage and prepare to do a little introspection here.

'Primary risk factors' increase your risk of having your first-ever episode. 'Secondary risk factors' increase the risk of it returning and of you becoming a long-term sufferer. To get right back from the edge and stay there, you must reduce your Risks.

Primary and secondary risk factors for LBP

Primary risk factors	Secondary risk factors
Loading – peak, cumulative and sustained	Previous back pain
Trauma	Lower level of back muscle endurance
Whole body vibration	Low mood – anxiety/ depression
Lower level of back muscle endurance	Stress
Work-related 'stress'	Obesity
Smoking	Passive coping/ catastrophising
Age – over 40	
Lower levels of physical fitness and activity	

The list is a little abstract in some cases. For example, obesity isn't a behaviour; you have to track the behaviours that contribute to the obesity and/or the behaviours that will reduce it. Working on these Risks can take time, and for some it's an ongoing challenge. Reducing your weight is one thing, but maintaining that new weight is a lifelong endeavour for many.

TOP TIP

Improving your mood if you're prone to anxiety is also a long-term project. That's why we run our Pain-Free & Confident Accelerator over 16 weeks (QR code in Chapter 16), to make sure you have all the tools to address these Risks.

Note that the single biggest risk factor for a new onset of LBP is having had it before. Don't worry – now you have this book, you can reduce that risk.

Achieving relief is usually the easy bit; Prevention requires you to dig deep over a longer period of time. Of course, all this measuring your Triggers, Aggravators and Risks should be associated with one of the other Essential Practices: Reduce (see Chapter 10).

CASE STUDY: Tracking improvements

Margaret had always felt that physical therapy was useful and that the exercises she was doing must be helping her, yet she hadn't made any progress with her sciatica over the last two years. She was still unable to play two days in a row.

Once she had her Backscore and started tracking it and some daily behaviours, she could see what helped her improve. Her Backscore went from 78 to 92 within two months. More importantly, she was finally able to play two days in a row, for the first time in three years.

Rule of Rehabilitation 1: Use it or lose it, but don't abuse it

Persistent pain is complex. You've seen some of the most obvious variables but there are other subtler ones. It is vitally important to have rules: in golf there are rules; in rehabilitation there are rules. Don't worry – there are only three of them for you to remember.

The road to recovery can be long and bumpy, and there can be dark times. The Rules of Rehabilitation are like your headlights; whenever you are in doubt, they will light your way. I wrote about this first rule in 1997 and have been living by it ever since. All my family and friends can recite this rule because I've been trotting it out multiple times a day for nearly thirty years.

In the short term, the Relief phase, this is the most important rule. It's always relevant, including throughout your journey back from the edge. Let's unpack this first Rule of Rehabilitation: Use it or lose it, but don't abuse it.

Use it or lose it...

I live in Scotland. It's a beautiful country with great people. In the winter, the weather isn't great for golf. Many golfers have a winter lay-off, then they dust off their clubs in the spring and head for the course. Many of them quickly develop pain. Why? Because over the winter months they lost capacity – they 'lost it'. They then exceeded their body's capacity in the spring, and it hurt.

When you don't do something for a while, you become deconditioned. You lose the ability to do that thing – or at least you lose the ability to do it safely. As you age, this deconditioning rate accelerates. If you could get away with a winter lay-off in your forties, you're less likely to get away with it in your seventies. This is a simple physiological fact – if you don't use your physical and mental capacities they will decline. That's the first part of Rule of Rehabilitation 1.

As you've seen from the Pain Equation (see Chapter 6), movement is hugely beneficial in dealing with pain (the MWP variable in the equation). This first part of Rule of Rehabilitation 1 reminds you of the importance of moving.

... But don't abuse it

Remember, if you do things that aggravate your pain it is unlikely to settle. You must either reduce the activity (Essential Practice 2, see Chapter 10), or find another way of doing it, such that it doesn't cause you pain. This is fundamental to your progress.

Sometimes there is a delay between doing something and the pain kicking in. Watch for this delayed example of 'abuse'. Whether the pain is worse at the time of doing something or later, this is all 'abuse'. I'm putting the rule in bold here because it is so important that you follow it:

Use it or lose it, but don't abuse it (UIOLIBDAI)

Summary

- There are two applications of 'measure': giving a fixed measure and tracking performance.

- The Backscore gives you a measure of the impact of your pain on your life.

- Your Functional Assessment guides you in many ways to make the right choices in your rehab.

- There are many things you can track to inform your progress – your Backscore, Aggravators, Triggers, Risks, Relievers, Preventers and variables of the Pain Equation.

- The first Rule of Rehabilitation is: Use it or lose it, but don't abuse it (UIOLIBDAI).

10
Essential Practice 2: Reduce

In this chapter, we'll be looking at the second Essential Practice: Reduce. You know from the Cliff of Pain (see Chapter 2) and the Pain Equation (see Chapter 6) that there are a number of things you can work on reducing. Measuring helps to keep track of your progress; it is important that you measure (track) the things you are reducing. In the early stages, you'll have to reduce Aggravators and Triggers. In the Prevention stage, you will have to reduce Risks.

Let's look to the two frameworks to see what can be reduced:

1. The Cliff of Pain

   - Aggravators

   - Triggers

   - Risks

2. The Pain Equation

   - Nociception

   - Negative thoughts

   - Attention to body part

Reduce nociception

How do you reduce nociception? Because you may not know whether you're dealing with nociceptive, nociplastic or even neurogenic pain, let pain be your guide.

Just reduce/modify activities that increase pain. (Remember that with inflammation, pain can be delayed.) This is reflected in the first Rule of Rehabilitation – Use it or lose it, but don't abuse it (see Chapter 9). If you keep doing things that cause nociceptive activity then the real origin of your pain will persist.

TOP TIP

To reduce nociceptive activity, you have to reduce the amount of stretching and loading you put on the injured disc.

As you now know, continued pain may not be due to ongoing nociception; it may be due to a sensitised nervous system (nociplastic pain). If you keep triggering those pain pathways to fire, it's likely that you will further reinforce them. Whether it's nociceptive, nociplastic or neuropathic pain, you're better to minimise it, otherwise you are likely to sensitise your nervous system and further reinforce your pain pathways.

Whatever your Aggravators are, you must reduce and/or modify them. As covered in Chapter 3, inflammation takes hours to build up – in the case of disc injuries, the inflammation often peaks on day two. You may need to look for those patterns where there's a delayed flare-up of pain. If you wake up in more pain, you should be considering what you have done differently over the previous two days (and consider your mattress). Resolve to do it differently, and track it.

Allow discs to heal and don't 'pick the scab'

If you have a problem with a disc – an annular tear, a bulge or a full prolapse – that disc needs to heal, and it can. Your immune system will cause an inflammatory response (which increases nociceptive activity, unfortunately). That inflammation is the first stage of healing. Specific cells, brought in by the inflammation, will eat away at the disc material that's in the wrong place, removing it over time.

The second stage is scar tissue formation. The tear in your disc needs to heal by the formation of new tissue. In the first few weeks, this new tissue is still weaker than it ultimately needs to be and is easily re-torn, therefore, you must avoid doing things that stretch it. If you stretch it, you're in danger of re-tearing it, causing more inflammation, and you're back to square one, which is painful. Remember, I call this 'picking the scab before it's ready to fall off'.

There are so many people that get stuck in this cycle that I have made a career out of the non-surgical rehabilitation of people with lumbar disc problems. In a way, they typify the whole field of LBP/sciatica rehabilitation – simple but not easy, but if you follow the rules you will succeed.

Again, if you'd like help achieving relief from this kind of pain, go to http://golf.painfreeandconfident. com/book-reader, where there's a section specifically on disc and nerve rehab, or scan the QR code.

Reduce sleep disruption

We're all aware that pain can disrupt our sleep. It turns out that disrupted sleep also increases our risk of pain. It's both a Risk and an Aggravator. In order to improve your sleep, there may be things you can reduce – for example, the use of screens close to bedtime. More on sleep in Chapter 12.

Reduce consumption of pro-inflammatory substances

Nicotine, ultra-processed foods (UPFs), sugar, food intolerances – these can all increase inflammation. One of my most listened-to podcast episodes is entitled, 'Can the coronavirus make my back pain or sciatica worse?' I was inspired to record this episode after being consulted by a number of patients who stated that the infection seemed to trigger an episode of their back pain or sciatica.

Admittedly, it could be a coincidence, but there's definitely a potential mechanism here. The virus – and other viruses – result in a body-wide inflammatory response. If you have nociceptors that are already sensitised, this widespread increase in inflammatory molecules could be enough to aggravate or trigger pain. Of course, this is not specific to LBP and sciatica. All persistent or recurrent pains can be triggered in this way. In one study, it was found that LBP sufferers with recent Covid-19 infections took longer to recover than those who didn't have a recent Covid-19 infection (Somma *et al.*, 2022).

Did you know that UPFs raise inflammation? So do high sugar levels. This is a huge issue for a lot of people. Reducing your intake of UPFs and sugar may be a life changer for you. Not just for your pain but for your general health and longevity.

Believe me, this isn't a side note for a minority of people. If you are consuming a substantial part of your calories as UPF, or you have a high sugar intake, this could be a huge contributor to your pain. Not just your back/sciatic pain, but all pains. According to many medical authorities, it'll also – almost certainly – shorten your life. This is one area you should seriously consider including in your daily tracking.

CASE STUDY: Reduce UPF, reduce pain

Gerry was struggling to achieve relief. He was carrying about 25 kilograms of excess body fat. When he reduced his consumption of UPF – even before the weight loss kicked in – his pain decreased markedly. He couldn't believe the difference.

His pain dropped from a daily average of 7/10 to 5/10 within three days of reducing his UPF consumption. This was the boost he needed to stick to his weight-loss plans.

Reducing or modifying Aggravators and Triggers

Reduce is relevant in the Relief phase, specifically with Triggers and Aggravators. It is also relevant in the Prevention phase in regard to risk factors and poor mood or stress, nociception and attention to body part. As you read this, you may want to refer back to the Pain Equation (see Chapter 6) – the understanding you gained there should inform this section.

I always say to my patients: 'If you want your back to get better, you have to stop doing the things that make it feel worse.' When I first said this, I thought it was too obvious and potentially offensive, but it may explain why you have failed to make progress. For me, it was a breakthrough – remember me, as a student, sitting for as long as I could before walking around at the back of the lecture room?

Stopping isn't always necessary, but, at the least, you have to reduce or modify your Aggravators and

Triggers so that they don't have that effect on you. If you choose not to do this, there's a real danger that you will not progress.

CASE STUDY: Putting challenges

Charlie had had persistent LBP for three years. It had built up gradually over the previous two years. He was still able to golf, with the use of painkillers, and usually played twice a week.

The biggest challenge for him was his putting; his particular stoop seemed to be the worst possible position for his back. That and brushing his teeth over the sink. Charlie was 6 foot 4 inches tall (201 cm), and putting with a standard-length putter. By using a longer putter and practising hip hinging when putting and brushing his teeth he solved the pain and regained confidence in his back.

Some Aggravators are easier to modify than others. Below are some common ones.

Sitting

This includes driving. When we conducted an audit of over 1,000 patients with LBP and sciatica, 78% of them found that sitting aggravated their pain. It certainly aggravated mine.

If you're in that group, you have a choice: reduce or modify? I'd recommend both, at least in the short term.

TOP TIP

If you're working at a desk for any length of time, I recommend a sit-stand desk or platform. This gives you options and enables you to vary the load. I have used a sit-stand desk for twenty-five years and it was a game changer for me, as it has been for many of our patients.

How should you modify? If your pain is worse the lower you sit, then I'd recommend you try to sit with your hips at least as high as your knees – preferably higher. Cars are mostly terrible for this. In most cars you'll find you are sitting with your knees higher than your hips. If you have head room to play with, get a folded-up towel or small cushion and put it under your bottom. The towel or cushion should not extend to your lower thighs; it's only for under your bottom. This will raise your hips relative to your knees.

If you'd like a fuller understanding of this and other dos and don'ts related to posture and bending, try the Rapid Relief Plan (see Chapter 3 for QR code).

Bending

Bending is a common Trigger and Aggravator. It's important that you determine whether it's bending forwards, backwards or (often) a combination of side-bending, rotation and forward bending. Whatever it is, you need to reduce or modify it – at least in the short term. Get your Functional Assessment (see Chapter 9) for further insights.

Sleeping

Often people struggle to sleep with LBP or sciatica. With sciatica, it's often because the pain builds up the longer you stay in a position – sometimes any position. With LBP it can be the same, but spasms of LBP on turning over are also quite common and may be indicative of instability (see Chapter 9).

I'm not saying you should reduce your sleep, but you may need to get creative. A few of my patients have had to sleep in two-hour bursts, then get up and move around and then go back to sleep. Staying in bed, their pain was escalating to the point that sleep was impossible. By walking around for twenty minutes they kept the pain levels down so that they could have three shifts of decent sleep a night, instead of watching the clock ticking by, wishing it was time to take their next dose of heavy-duty painkillers.

Walking

Walking is valuable to your overall health and – unless you're going to use a buggy – it's essential for golf.

If you can't find a way of walking that doesn't reduce your pain, you will have to minimise it, at least in the short term.

TOP TIP

If you have pain while walking, try shortening your stride.

Coughing and sneezing

Coughing and sneezing can be a nightmare – especially sneezing, which involves a powerful contraction of your abdominal and pelvic muscles. This results in a high strain on your muscles and discs. If you have a grumbly/bulging/prolapsed disc, it can be painful indeed. The below advice related to sneezing is particularly relevant if you have – or think you may have – a disc problem:

- If you feel a sneeze coming on and you're lying down, stay lying down. Do not sit up, whatever you do.

- If you are sitting and you feel a sneeze coming on, try to slide your bottom forward in the seat but keep your lower back arched so that you're getting as close to horizontal as possible.

- If you are already standing up, try to lean on a wall with the hand opposite your sciatic pain (if you have sciatica) and lift that foot of the sciatica side off the floor.

143

I don't want to freak you out, but I've known a few sufferers over the years who have gone from a low-grade grumbly disc to a large disc prolapse by sneezing. Try to remember this.

TOP TIP

Some people find that pressing their tongue against the back of their upper front teeth stops a sneeze from happening.

Golfing

I'm not a golf coach (I collaborate with golfing experts), but my advice comes from being a pain coach. If you are playing golf in such a way or with such frequency that you are aggravating your pain, you need to reduce that: swing less often or swing differently.

On our Pain-Free & Confident Accelerator (see QR code in Chapter 16), we include a session with a golf swing coach early in the programme. We like to keep you on the course but swinging in such a way that you aren't jeopardising your recovery (applying Rule of Rehabilitation 1). In Chapter 15, we'll cover swing modifications in more detail.

CASE STUDY: Golf without painkillers

Jose had been using ibuprofen and paracetamol before every round of golf for the last two years. It enabled him to get round with only mild pain. His pain wasn't getting any better and sometimes would flare up so that he would miss weeks of golf at a time.

By sticking to twelve holes at a time and golfing without painkillers and anti-inflammatories, only playing two rounds a week, and sticking to the Rules of Rehabilitation, he finally started making progress. Now he is golfing eighteen holes four times a week without flare-ups (or medication).

TRY IT YOURSELF

Make a list of all the things you could reduce. Pick one or two that you think will be most impactful, and start with those.

Summary

- Reducing Risks, Aggravators and Triggers is key.

- Reducing some variables in the Pain Equation is another lever to pull.

- Going further upstream to reduce behaviours that impact the variables in the Pain Equation and the Cliff of Pain is helpful too.

- Reducing golf may be necessary in the short term.

11
Essential Practice 3: Relax

This chapter is all about relaxing. It isn't only about reducing stress and threat, although that's a big part of it. If that's all it was about, I could simply have packaged it up under the reduce practice. Relaxing isn't just the opposite of being stressed, just as being healthy isn't just the absence of illness – it's much more than that.

Relaxing: More than just the removal of stress and anxiety

Many people struggle with the idea that what's going on in their mind can perpetuate their pain. You may like to think body and mind are separate issues and the pain is all in your back or leg. Having read Part

147

3, you may have accepted – in principle – that pain is modified by the brain and spinal cord, but when it comes down to it, you're still convinced that it's all about your back.

Don't forget the story of the builder with the nail through his boot (see Chapter 6) or underestimate the power of the mind in maintaining your pain. Don't forget that catastrophising is a Risk for persistent pain but not for first-time pain. The nervous system has a big role to play in moving you into persistent pain and keeping you there.

It may be that stress is a small contributor to your pain, but it may also be the missing key. You know the saying, 'A chain is only as strong as its weakest link'; you don't want weaknesses, because those are the silent risks pushing you back towards the edge. Your weaknesses will undermine your progress. They become your biggest threat of relapse because those are the areas you haven't been addressing head on.

Reducing threat

'Perceived threat' is more closely correlated with levels of pain than actual tissue damage. If you think something is likely to lead to pain, it's highly likely that it will. Inversely, if you can convince yourself that it won't, then it is less likely to. If you can distract yourself effectively, then it's even less likely to (remember attention to body part in the Pain

Equation?), especially if that distraction is enjoyable and with someone you like being with.

One of the big challenges here is movements that have previously triggered painful episodes. You are likely to perceive those as threatening, and yet they are often movements you want to be able to do. Putting may be a good example of this, or bending over to tee up your ball or to get your ball out of the hole. This is an example of the third rule in play (we'll come to that soon).

If there are movements that are important to you, you have to factor them into your rehab. How do you reduce the perceived threat and build yourself back up to the point that you can do these activities again? By following the three Rules of Rehabilitation.

Reducing stress

I've come to think of stress as imperceptible threats or fears that you haven't necessarily consciously considered fully. For some people, that may be uncertainty over the security of their job, their income, a relationship or their future health. These are present in many people but are often not articulated. Although you may not have articulated them clearly to yourself or someone else, they are still there. These are properly known as 'stressors' (things that cause stress). Stress is what you experience, whereas a stressor is the causative agent.

Some people think and talk themselves into a state of stress frequently. These people are termed 'anxious'. Anxiety is fear about potential future events, and this fear about the future leads to stress. If you stand over the ball convinced that you're going to play a poor shot, then you are an anxious golfer.

The best way to reduce stress is to reduce anxiety. That may require some form of counselling, such as cognitive behavioural therapy. There are a number of other ways to reduce the impact of stress on your body and nervous system. Here are a few you may want to incorporate into your daily practice.

- **Massage:** Massage is extremely effective at dropping you into a relaxed state. It's great for stimulating mechanoreceptors, which help to block nociceptive input (see Chapter 6). Massage can help in at least two ways with reducing pain.

- **Meditation:** Meditation has been shown repeatedly to lower stress levels and improve focus – useful for pain and golf.

- **Sleeping well:** I cover this in Chapter 12.

- **Moving often (especially when under pressure):** Movement is a tremendous way to reduce stress. The quickest way to change your mental state is to change your physical state.

- **Reducing relationship issues:** It's important to recognise that relationships are the greatest source of stress in most people's lives. Fortunately, they are also the greatest source of joy for many. That's where the 'Enjoy' practice comes (see Chapter 14).

- **Positive affirmations:** Having a negative outlook is one of the variables in The Pain Equation (see Chapter 6) that will increase your pain. You need to develop the opposite. This particularly relates to your back but it's true for all aspects of life. Remember, your brain doesn't differentiate between threats related to your back and other general threats. The more threat or stress your brain perceives, the more it will augment your pain. Developing a positive affirmation can directly reduce your pain. Here are some to try: 'My back is strong', 'My back is resilient', 'My back is getting stronger', 'My back and I are getting stronger'. Choose one that resonates with you or craft your own.

- **Positive visualisation:** In our Pain-Free & Confident Accelerator programme (see QR code in Chapter 16), we teach participants a particular type of positive visualisation. If you haven't stood on the tee and visualised your ball flying, landing and rolling to where you want it to be, you are unusual. Most top golfers use visualisation, and it can be applied to becoming pain-free and confident (we'll cover this more in Chapter 13).

Stress and my pain

Do you think having a disagreement with a family member might be enough to trigger your LBP? It has been for me on more than one occasion. Just a few months ago, I had a run-in with a close family member, someone I love. We separated without having resolved the disagreement.

That evening, I decided to do a little yoga – which is a common practice for me in the evenings. I was doing something I have done thousands of times before – sitting with my legs straight out in front of me and leaning forwards over them, reaching past my toes. Twang! I had a small but obvious spasm of pain in my lower back. Twenty years ago, I would have panicked, but this time I knew what was going on. This pain was purely triggered by negative thinking and my past history of LBP (which was extensive, remember). What did I do? I did some breathing to calm my mind and repeated the same yoga pose – this time, no pain. Because I had not damaged my back in this position, this was not nociceptive pain – it was entirely nociplastic.

I have had many instances of pain being triggered by stress over the last thirty years. In fact, it's the most common Trigger for me. Sitting a lot can still be a Trigger too, but I find that easier to reduce than stress. Have a think about your pain. Is it worse when life is against you? Is it worse when you are stressed? Time to work on that.

Breathwork

Breathing is something we all do, and we do it a lot: around 22,000 times per day. It turns out many of us do it poorly. There have been some great books written on this subject recently. In this chapter we are focused on relaxing, and there's certainly a lot you can do with your breath to improve this practice. You can also use breathing to optimise for performance – many tour golfers do so, both to optimise their power production for distance and to calm the mind for the pressure putts.

The parasympathetic nervous system

Recent evidence suggests that people with persistent pain have a poorer functioning parasympathetic nervous system. People who are anxious often have an imbalance between their sympathetic and parasympathetic nervous systems (PNS) – the parts of your nervous system that control background activities such as digestion, heart rate and sweating. You may have heard about the sympathetic nervous system being involved in the fear/flight/fight response. The parasympathetic system is more about rest and digest. It helps to down-regulate pain too. If this system isn't working as well, what can you do to train your PNS to perform better?

Before I answer that, how do we measure the strength of your PNS? A fairly accessible way is to assess your heart rate variability (HRV) – a measure of how your heart rate varies. 'Heart rate' tells us how many times your heart beats in a certain period. HRV is about the variation in time between beats. Typically, the time between heartbeats is less as you breathe in and more as you breathe out. A higher HRV indicates that your PNS is in good shape; a lower HRV indicates that it isn't.

A word of warning: HRVs differ significantly between people and it's pointless comparing with others. There are a number of wearables, including many smartwatches, that track HRV. You really need a month of tracking to get a baseline of what is normal for you. There are also devices available that enable you to train your HRV through breathwork, thereby boosting your PNS and – potentially – reducing pain. Again, many tour pros are using this technology.

How to breathe to relax

In short, it's important to have a long exhale to push you towards a more relaxed state. Make sure you breathe in through your nose. The physiological sigh has been promoted as the quickest way to put your body and mind into a rest and recovery state, moving you from anxious to calm. There are other practices that help, such as box breathing and yoga nidra.

Here's how to practise the physiological sigh: Take a sharp breath in through your nose, immediately followed by another breath in through the nose, so it's like a double sniff. Breathe out through the mouth, making your exhale long and slow, through pursed lips. You could do three or four of these in a row, but even one will have an immediate impact. I've shared this with many golfers, and most of them have found it useful.

TRY IT YOURSELF

I have to credit former PGA golf coach Gary Nicol for this one. Holding your breath as you play a shot is not the optimal way to swing. You generate more power on the exhale.

My practice now is to breathe in as I begin to pull the clubhead back and start to exhale as I begin my downswing. It removes a lot of tension from the body for the follow-through, reducing stress on your body, including your lower back. Many of our golfers have found this makes for an easier, less stressful downswing and follow-through.

Summary

- Relaxing isn't just about reducing stress – it should be more proactive than that.

- There are many ways to relax, including massage, meditation, sleeping well, moving often, reducing relationship issues, positive affirmations and positive visualisation.

- Breathwork is one of the most powerful and immediate ways to reduce stress and pain.

12
Essential Practice 4: Optimise

In this chapter we're going to look at the optimise practice. There are many things you could be optimising and we will cover the most important in the context of the Cliff of Pain (see Chapter 2) and the Pain Equation (see Chapter 6). As you are a golfer, and golf exerts a particular load on the lower back, let's start with loading.

Acute-to-chronic workload ratio

I'm not sure when I first became aware of Tim Gabbett's work (https://gabbettperformance.com.au/profile). Like all top researchers, he has collaborated with many other researchers, so it's important to acknowledge that this is not the work of one man on his own. A quick Google will show you that the acute-to-chronic workload ratio (ACWR) is associated with him more than any other researcher. Although Tim works closely with a lot of elite-level national and international sports teams, I see no reason that his ratio shouldn't be as applicable to the untrained as it is to the highly trained. He was kind enough to reply to a speculative email I wrote to him about this, and that was his view too.

What does the ACWR tell us?

The ratio compares the workload performed in the last week with the average week over the previous four weeks (Gabbett, 2016). Again, we're back to acute meaning short term and chronic meaning long term – although in this case they are using one week and four weeks respectively (rather than less than six weeks and more than twelve weeks in the world of pain – see Chapter 6).

What does the ACWR state?

Before we come to that, let's define 'workload' because this is relevant to LBP. One of the Risks for LBP is loading, of which there are three types: peak, cumulative and sustained (see Chapter 5). Interestingly, chronic workload is a similar concept to cumulative loading. Swinging a golf club repeatedly definitely qualifies as cumulative loading. For many of us, a full swing can qualify as peak load.

Loading can be sitting, standing, running, carrying, lifting, golfing and so on. Gravity is exerting a load on us all the time, even when we are lying down. Some people cannot lie in bed for longer than their normal duration; they simply can't enjoy a weekend lie-in because the pain worsens the longer they stay in bed. Is this due to tissues being tired out by being kept in one position for a prolonged period – sustained loading? It could be due to the build-up of inflammation too (see Chapter 3).

Back to the ACWR. It states that the risk of injury goes up if the ratio is well in excess of 1.3. That means that if you do 30% more than you're used to doing (ACWR = 1.3), your risk of injury goes up because you've overloaded the tissues. The highest risk of injury is with a high ACWR, ie >1.5. This would mean you did 50% more workload in the last week than you did in the average of the previous four weeks.

Tim's follow-up paper in 2020 indicates that load should not be regarded as the only predictor of risk. Other factors such as low volume/quality of sleep, work and relationship stressors can also increase the risk. Much like pain itself, injury is not solely due to overloading. In fact, risk of injury is determined by multiple factors.

What does this mean in the world of golf? There are three common scenarios I have seen:

1. **Golf trips:** This seems obvious. You're used to playing once a week. It seems like a great idea to go on a golf trip and play four rounds in three days. Your ACWR in this scenario would be 4:1 (ie 4.0), which is enormous and results in a clear risk of injury.

2. **Recent retirement:** You've been scaling down work gradually and managed to play two rounds of golf a week for the last six months. Now you're fully retired and you hit three rounds in your first week of retirement. Your ACWR is 3:2 (ie 1.5), which is high and increases your risk of injury.

3. **Spring start-up:** You've only played golf occasionally through the winter, averaging once every two weeks (that's nine holes per week, based on a full eighteen). As soon as the season starts, you hit two rounds in the first week. Your ACWR is 36:9 (ie 4.0) – a very high risk of injury.

Age

Another important factor to consider here is age. The older you are, the slower your tissues are to adapt. If you have a lay-off in your thirties, you can probably swing without much fear in the spring. A five-month lay-off in your seventies should result in a gradual build-up. It's likely that as we age, the ACWR window narrows. That is to say you need to be closer to 1 from both ends. My guess is that for those over seventy, you want an ACWR of 0.9 to 1.2. The ACWR is science's ratification of my second Rule of Rehabilitation.

Rule of Rehabilitation 2: Start low and build slow

For a while, you have to reduce or avoid certain activities. When you reintroduce them – or start anything new – you should start low and build slow (SLABS). This second Rule of Rehabilitation is consistent with the ACWR and pain science. In the field of pain rehabilitation/management this is referred to as 'graded exposure'. Whichever type, or combination of types, of pain you have – nociceptive (due to what's going on in your back), neuropathic (due to direct irritation of spinal nerves) or nociplastic (learnt pain) – graded exposure is appropriate.

CASE STUDY: Too much too soon

Euan had a disc prolapse that caused nociceptive pain via inflammation in his L4L5. He also had neuropathic sciatic pain, as the disc prolapse was irritating his L5 nerve root (which gave branches to the sciatic nerve). He had been in pain for six months, and noticed his pain was worse when stressed or sleep-deprived (nociplastic pain). He had fallen off the Cliff of Pain a few times, always because he'd been feeling that little bit better and had virtually doubled his activity in one day.

By following the SLABS rule, he was finally able to avoid flare-ups and recover fully.

Optimise movement and loading

You're now acquainted with the first two Rules of Rehabilitation:

1. Use it or lose it but don't abuse it (UIOLIBDAI)

2. Start low and build slow (SLABS)

These rules are your guiding principles in movement and loading.

Your body has the wonderful capacity to adapt and grow stronger – of course, this diminishes as we age, but it's still possible in old age to grow stronger. There are two phases to strengthening tissues: you have to stress the body to stimulate the response, but it's during the rest days that the body builds strength. There needs to be the stimulus and the opportunity for growth. If it's all stimulus, there is no growth – just fatigue and tissue breakdown. If it's all rest and no stimulus, then you lose it. The ACWR will be a guideline for you to reduce the risk of injury.

Note that in the early stages of recovering from pain, and the ongoing stages if you have nociplastic pain, it's probably pain rather than the tissues' capacity for growth that will be the limiting factor on your progression. Although we're talking about movement and loading in a mechanical sense, you have to remember that movement and loading can also lead to both nociceptive input and a reaction within a sensitised nervous system (the consequences of nociplastic changes). How do you work this out? Simply follow the Rules of Rehabilitation – that's what they're for:

- Move often in ways that don't cause pain – this could just be walking.

- Use a variety of postures and movements.

- Build up load gradually and keep progressing (that's how to get stronger and build your confidence).

- Take part in movements that relate to your long-term goal (so long as they don't increase your pain).

Optimise sitting

In our clinic, an audit of over 1,000 LBP and sciatica patients revealed that around 78% find that sitting is an Aggravator. If you'd like guidance on how you can sit to minimise pain, try the free Rapid Relief Plan (see Chapter 3 for QR code).

Optimise bending

Bending is a common Aggravator too; this is a big factor for many sufferers. There's more than one way to bend. You need to bend in such a way that you're not aggravating your pain. We like to teach people how to bend optimally, ie in a way that avoids pain but is also the most mechanically efficient and powerful way to bend. I'll talk about hip hinging in Chapter 15.

Optimise golfing

We can't leave out your golf swing. You should work out whether it's the swing or the walking or pulling your trolley that's the Aggravator. Once you've done that, you may need to modify or reduce your swing in the short term. You then need to optimise it for the result you're looking for – swinging pain-free and with confidence, I imagine. (We cover swing modifications in Chapter 15.)

Optimise standing and walking

Golfers with pain standing or walking are generally harder to help than those with sitting problems – sitting isn't necessary for golf but standing and walking are. Much like your golf swing, it's useful if you can work out which phase of the walking step is a problem. Is it the heel-strike, or is walking uphill or downhill worse? All of this will influence the modifications you might make to help.

Changes that are often helpful are shortening your stride or simply walking more carefully. Or using light abdominal bracing while walking – you can initiate this by trying to walk taller. This will get your abdominal muscles to work to stabilise your spine better.

TOP TIP

Some golfers find a change of shoes helpful, particularly with a more cushioned sole.

For me, optimising movement and loading means doing so in such a way that I'm increasing my back's – and my whole body's – capacity to deal with load. I have a maxim: 'In nature, nothing stands still – it's either growing or dying.' You want to slowly (SLABS) increase your capacity to deal with load, otherwise there's a good chance you'll be getting weaker (nothing stands still).

It's totally your decision, but I'd recommend measuring this. Track it over time. At the least, try to ensure your capacity for dealing with load is not decreasing. The most obvious measure for a golfer is – can you play as many holes as you used to, without being more tired?

Month to month, I track my load-bearing capacity and strength in the gym. Can I lift as much weight cumulatively in a training session as I could last month?

Ideally, I would lift more from year to year. I heard a podcast interview with Arnold Schwarzenegger in 2023 – in his mid-seventies. He said, 'The older I get, the harder I have to work.' You may not have any aspiration to achieve his muscularity (and neither do I), but he makes an important point.

Optimise other activities

What else do you need to optimise for? Gardening? Lifting grandchildren? Curling? Make sure you factor in all your ambitions and that you relate (the next Essential Practice) your day-to-day activities to that long-term goal.

Other benefits of movement

Movement improves blood circulation, bringing in nutrients for healing and washing away the waste products. It also moves inflammation along. One reason an arthritic joint feels worse after sitting for a while is that the inflammation has built up. Conversely, it feels better for a little gentle movement. The same goes for your back.

Movement also boosts mood, especially if it's more vigorous or sustained. You produce natural painkillers – endorphins and endocannabinoids – when you exercise. These are powerful painkillers, suppressing the pain pathways. Movement – so long as it's not delaying healing or triggering your pain pathways (don't abuse it) – is one of your most powerful relieving tactics.

Optimise nutrition

There are two main points here:

1. Being overweight is a risk factor for persistent LBP.
2. Certain foods promote inflammation, which will increase nociceptive activity.

Being overweight

If you have a large belly, do you think that puts more strain on your lower back? It probably does. To be fair, so long as you gained that weight gradually, your back may have been able to adapt to the extra weight and essentially get stronger. We don't know that the extra load is the main driver of pain, but it may be a factor.

What do we know? We know that carrying excess body fat results in more inflammation in the body, and inflammation increases nociception. Reducing weight (body fat) is likely to reduce pain. This may be a new idea for you, but it's widely written about in medical research. When you gain fat, you don't gain more fat cells (adipocytes); the adipocytes you have swell up. When they do so, they produce pro-inflammatory cytokines. These chemicals – such as Interleukin-6 – drive inflammation around the body, thereby contributing to pain and a whole host of other things you'd rather not have (like heart disease).

Pro-inflammatory foods

Some people have food sensitivities and intolerances that can cause more inflammation in their systems. This would drive more pain. Others have low-grade allergies to some foods, and this would certainly also result in raised levels of inflammation. If you suspect you may have an intolerance, you could consult a functional medicine practitioner.

TRY IT YOURSELF

If you think you may have a food sensitivity, intolerance or allergy, try eliminating the food for a while to see whether your pain diminishes. Does your pain increase when you reintroduce the food?

CASE STUDY: The impact of diet and nutrition on pain

Susan had been told she had a disc bulge that was aggravating her sciatic nerve. She had had this pain for six months and it wasn't budging. She was considering surgery. In discussion, it was clear that her pain varied quite a lot, although there wasn't a clear pattern. She had been overweight for many years and struggled to lose weight.

Out of desperation, she decided to try a low-carbohydrate diet. Within two days of starting the diet she had lost 1.5 kilograms (probably nearly entirely water). More impressively, her average pain level had dropped from 6/10 to 3/10 and her most severe pains from 8/10 to 5/10.

This was clearly not due to weight loss. Later, a genetic test revealed that she was likely to be slightly sensitive to gluten. By going on a low-carb diet she had eliminated nearly all gluten from her diet. Was that the reason for her dramatic pain reduction? We can't be sure, but I think so.

The principle of this case study applies to all areas we are covering here. Until you try to make some of the recommended changes – and measure their impact – you won't know how much better you could feel.

Optimise sleep

Poor sleep (lack of it or poor-quality sleep) directly influences levels of pain. Obviously, if you're in pain at night, that's going to result in poor-quality sleep, but poor sleep is an 'independent risk factor' for persistent pain; it's not listed in the table of risk factors in Chapter 5 as most research studies into LBP didn't assess for this. Poor sleep is definitely going to aggravate your pain if you're not getting a good full night's sleep – for whatever reason.

A scientific review of the relationship between sleep and pain concluded 'sleep impairments reliably predict new incidents and exacerbations of chronic pain' (Finan, Goodin and Smith, 2013). While some of this is to do with the central nervous system (brain and spinal cord), there is also evidence that poor sleep quality and quantity sensitises your nociceptors, making them more likely to 'fire'. One study involving rats demonstrated that disrupted sleep resulted in increased sensitivity of the nociceptors (Kim *et al.*, 2019). (It's difficult to do these sorts of studies on humans so the poor rats take our place.)

If poor sleep increases nociception and sensitises the pain pathways, and pain leads to poor sleep, you can easily get stuck in a vicious circle: poor sleep leading to more pain, which leads to poorer sleep, which leads to more pain, and so on.

Because good sleep is so incredibly important to recovery, I will often recommend that patients use effective pain relief at night (you should consult your physician about the use of pain-relieving medication). The need for sleep overrides everything.

Sleep is so important that we include a tutorial with a sleep coach in our Pain-Free & Confident Accelerator (see QR code in Chapter 16).

Exercises for prevention

Exercises for prevention is a big topic. Let me make a few points first. Always stick to the Rules of Rehabilitation. Most notably, if an exercise increases your pain, you shouldn't be doing it – at least, not now.

Lack of physical activity is a risk factor for LBP. Doing more physical activity – of nearly any type – is likely to reduce your risk. As a golfer, it's likely you get plenty of walking. If you're having to use a buggy, please try to walk as much as you can, while following the Rules of Rehabilitation.

Which exercises are not likely to prevent persistent LBP? Stretching exercises (if you don't know why by now, go back to Chapter 4). As a golfer, you put your spine under quite a lot of load and it's important to prepare it for that. One of the best ways is by swinging a golf club.

What about swing trainer aids? Fine, so long as you don't break the Rules of Rehabilitation. Nearly everyone I've met has broken the SLABS rule when they first bought a swing trainer aid. Admittedly, nearly everyone I meet has LBP, so it's a skewed population.

What do I do? Lack of back muscle endurance is a risk factor for persistent pain, so you need to address that.

Is that the same as core exercises? They are similar.

Is there compelling evidence that one exercise, eg Pilates or a combination of exercises are better than all the others? No. There's a lot of research in this space, but there isn't an obvious winner.

TRY IT YOURSELF

Go back to the Cliff of Pain image you drew for yourself in Chapter 2. Look at your risk factors and ask yourself what you could optimise to improve on these. Write down your answers and add them to a spreadsheet on which you can track (measure) your progress.

Scan the QR code in Chapter 3 for access to videos of the exercises I start all our golfers on. The idea with these exercises is to give you the best bang for your buck with the least risk. I recommend you aim for a programme that takes you about eight to ten minutes a day and do them every day. It's much easier to maintain a daily habit than it is to maintain a three-times-a-week habit.

Summary

- The ACWR is an important framework to avoid overloading and injuring your back.

- The second Rule of Rehabilitation is: Start low and build slow (SLABS) – it is the application of the ACWR.

- You can optimise the different variables in the Pain Equation and the Cliff of Pain, and their upstream behaviours.

- Preventer exercises can optimise your back's strength and endurance.

13
Essential Practice 5: Relate

This practice is about connecting everything you do to your goal of getting back from the edge. It's also about the stories you tell yourself and how to use those to improve your situation. There are two definitions of 'relate' that we need to explore.

1. Relate: To tell a story or describe a series of events

Do you hear that voice inside your head? The one that is always there, offering its opinion. What does it usually tell you about your back? Is it worrying about the next time you golf? Is it telling you your back is weak, that it's only a matter of time before your next episode?

You may not be an out-and-out catastrophiser, but after many episodes of LBP it's totally understandable if you're expecting the worst. Any negative self-talk jeopardises the achievement of your long-term goal. This is the equivalent of standing on the tee and thinking, 'I better not put it in the water.' Your brain doesn't recognise negatives. All it hears is 'put it in the water'. If there is any negative self-talk, it's time to change the record.

Change your story

This practice is all about Rule of Rehabilitation 3: Keep the end in mind. Once you have defined your SMART goal (one that is specific, measurable, achievable, relevant and time-bound), you have to start telling yourself that story. If you can picture yourself achieving that goal – visualise yourself – then you are far more likely to achieve your goal.

I'd like you to describe a series of events (relate them) in the future that fit with your SMART goal. Goals help you to define the future you would like. To achieve that goal, you have to see the steps that will take you to it, and it helps if you visualise yourself taking those steps. By mapping out those steps and seeing yourself take them, you are far more likely to do so. That is a scientific fact.

When you tell yourself the story, you will be changing your self-image from 'I'm a golfer with a weak back' to something like 'I have a strong pain-free lower back

I have confidence in'. To achieve that, you might want to use this phrase: 'I'm the sort of person who…'.

If you are to become a golfer with a strong pain-free lower back you can have confidence in, then what sort of person do you need to be?

- The sort of person who consistently does Preventer exercises

- The sort of person who diligently reduces their risk factors

- The sort of person who sticks to the Rules of Rehabilitation

These are all a bit theoretical. You need to personalise this visualisation process.

Self-image statements

Maybe your SMART goal is: 'It's 1 September and I am just finishing my fourth round of golf in five days. My lower back is pain-free and I'm confident it will remain so.'

To achieve this, here are some possible statements related to self-image:

- I'm the sort of person who has completed Preventer exercises six days out of seven for the previous four months.

- I'm the sort of person who has kept carbs to a minimum and lost 10 kilograms of fat in the previous four months.

- I'm the sort of person who has steadily built stability and strength in their lower back over the previous three months.

TRY IT YOURSELF

Every morning, visualise yourself completing that long-term SMART goal, then visualise the steps you are going to take today that will take you one day closer to achieving that goal. The whole thing could take you ninety seconds.

From the self-image statements above, now visualise yourself, doing your Preventer exercises, eating meals with low-carbohydrate content and doing strengthening exercises in the gym.

How to visualise

Involve as many of your senses as possible (some may not be relevant to the visualisation you're trying to have):

- Seeing

- Hearing

- Smelling

- Touching
- Tasting
- Kinaesthetic sense (how your body feels as it moves)

Feel those sensations as you visualise yourself completing those steps. This is the way to maximise the chances that you will actually complete the necessary steps today. Most top sportspeople visualise their success, and they do it vividly. You've probably done it on the golf course – visualised your ball landing mid-fairway and rolling on 30 yards to come to rest, with an easy wedge into the green.

2. Relate: To find or show connection between two things

The other – more common – meaning of 'relate' ties in totally with the third Rule of Rehabilitation: Keep the end in mind. You must ensure that much of what you do relates to your goal. It's no use having a goal but doing things that don't in any way relate to it.

Play golf

You must play golf. At the least, you must swing a club, even if it's just chipping and putting. Do whatever your back can manage without aggravating your pain, ie apply the first two rules.

The longer you go without playing, the more deconditioned you become for golf (use it or lose it). If you've
come to associate golf with pain, then the longer you
go without playing, the more sensitised your pain is
likely to become to golfing (remember how sensitised
I became to sitting by avoiding it). For some golfers,
this is a big hurdle.

It's what you want to do, it's what you would love
to do, but you've had so many episodes triggered
by golfing that you are fearful. As you reduce those
risk factors you will be moving back from the edge.
You won't be so easily triggered. Stick to the Rules of
Rehabilitation and the six Essential Practices and you
will get there. Go for it.

Rule of Rehabilitation 3:
Keep the end in mind

Remember the Fear Avoidance Model (see Chapter 5)?
One of the big mistakes I made in my twenties was that I
avoided sitting as much as possible. Way past the point of
healing. I managed to remain pain-free a lot of the time,
but I was totally intolerant of sitting for many years.

Most people sit quite a bit of the time. There are lots of
social activities that tend to involve sitting:

- Dining with friends and family
- Travelling to visit friends or family

- Cinema and theatre
- Watching sports
- Desk work

My mistake was that I didn't think about what I wanted in the long term; instead, I was focused on avoiding pain. As a result, my pain was frequently triggered by sitting. I couldn't confidently go out for dinner. My wife was often frustrated that I would judge a restaurant on its chairs rather than its food. I couldn't drive long distances two days in a row. I had to buy a hydraulic desk so that I could stand to work, rather than be forced to sit (I bought my first one in 1997).

Be clear about what it is that you want – that is what you have to optimise for. A lot of your day-to-day activities *must* relate to your goal. This is why I always want you to stay swinging a club, while adhering to the other Rules of Rehabilitation. If you want to play golf into your nineties, then keep swinging frequently.

Looking at the Rules of Rehabilitation together

If you haven't already, you should set a SMART goal. Here's an example: 'It's 1 October and I can play three rounds of eighteen holes in a week without pain and without fear of pain.'

The double benefit of this third Rule of Rehabilitation is that it reminds you what you're doing all of this for. It ensures that you will be optimising for your desired outcome and not just 'getting better' – which is far too vague to keep you accountable. How will you know that you're making progress towards your SMART goal? Because you'll be practising the first of the six Essential Practices: Measure.

Let's take a look at those practices now and see the three Rules of Rehabilitation applied together. We'll use teeing up your ball as an example.

Being able to bend over freely and painlessly to tee your ball up may be one of your golfing goals. Here I'm assuming that you have the capacity to regain the physical range of movement and strength required to get down to the ball and back up again. You may not have this range of movement currently if you've avoided this activity for a long time. Let's assume it is physically possible, were it not for pain.

Following the Rules of Rehabilitation:

- **Keep the end in mind:** It's vitally important that you practise the things that you ultimately want to do. If you don't, they are likely to remain hazardous for you. Remember that I avoided sitting for years (as much as possible) and so it was always a Trigger for me. Now I can slump with the best of them, should I choose to. If you don't practise teeing the ball up, and it's been a Trigger or Aggravator for you, then it's unlikely you'll regain this capacity.

- **Use it or lose it, but don't abuse it:** Do the movement to the limit of your capacity, without pain. Modify the movement to get lower – experiment.

  If it's painful to even start the movement, back off and use visualisation instead. This is an effective way to relax your mind. Imagine yourself doing the activity. See yourself teeing the ball up, unhindered by pain or restriction. Once you have frequently visualised this activity over a week or so (without triggering pain), go back and try the movement again. Amazingly, just visualising the movement can desensitise the brain's pain pathways.

- **Start low and build slow:** As you are able to, slowly build up the movement progressively, only increasing by small increments. Whatever you want to achieve, you have to prioritise. If teeing up the ball is important, practise this movement several times a day.

The same process can be followed for other movements or activities.

Summary

- There are two types of relating: the stories you tell yourself and tying everything back to your long-term goal.

- Have a long-term SMART goal. Visualise it daily – and how you're going to move towards that goal today.

- The third Rule of Rehabilitation is: Keep the end in mind (KTEIM). It ties your behaviours to your long-term goals.

- You should be playing as much golf as the first two Rules of Rehabilitation permit.

14
Essential Practice 6: Enjoy

This chapter is about the last of the six Essential Practices: Enjoy. Although I've written the least on this practice, you shouldn't underestimate it. It can be a powerful antidote to pain.

Enjoy your relationships

Let's start with relationships. You'll remember that negative thoughts are one of the variables that increase pain (see Chapter 6). You'll also remember that the psychosocial factors are the strongest of the Risks for moving from acute to chronic LBP (see Chapter 7) – 'social' means relationships.

Is it possible that relationships are the greatest source of stress in your life? I know they have been in mine (thankfully, they're the greatest source of pleasure too).

Reduce negative relationships

There are established neurobiological mechanisms connecting pain and stress (go back to The Pain Equation in Chapter 6 to remind yourself, if you need to). It may be necessary for you to improve your relationships to reduce your pain. Sometimes, if the other person won't work with you to improve the relationship, it's necessary to end the relationship to reduce physical pain (never mind the psychological pain). This is true for all relationships: family, friends and work.

I am neither a mental health professional nor a counsellor. There are legions of good books about family, social and business relationships. You can start by reading some of those, but, as I stated earlier, reading is not enough. You have to do something differently if you're going to improve your relationships. Knowledge is simply not enough; you must act.

Once you've decided how you're going to act, come back to this book. I'm going to talk about habit changing soon, which will help you to incorporate the required changes into how you relate to others. This will hopefully also change how they relate to you.

Enjoy positive relationships

Just as negative relationships increase pain, so positive relationships can reduce it. Go out with your golfing friends. If you can't walk that distance, then drive a buggy. If you can't swing due to pain but you can walk, then walk around. At the least, meet them for a chat after the round. Enjoying positive relationships is one of the most powerful things you can do to reduce the risk and impact of persistent pain.

Who makes you laugh? Who makes you feel good? Spend more time with those people. Your pain will be lower when you're with them, I promise.

There's a broader point here too. Remember the 'attention to body part' variable (see Chapter 6)? The more attention you give your LBP, the worse it will feel. Enjoying yourself moves your attention away from your pain and that reduces it. Anyone for golf?

CASE STUDY: The pain of a bad relationship

Mac had been in pain for years. He was down to nine holes a week. The consultant neurosurgeon said his symptoms matched his MRI – disc bulge at L4-L5 on the left. He had resisted surgery but tried just about everything else.

Then his wife of thirty years told him she was leaving; the kids were grown up and she had had enough. He agreed. They had both suffered enough through years of a dysfunctional marriage. They separated quickly. Within a month, his pain was 60% better and it continued to improve.

Mac is convinced nothing else changed, just the stress of his relationship reduced dramatically. Up until then, he had refused to believe that stress could be a factor in his pain. Go figure.

TRY IT YOURSELF

Write out a list of all the people you enjoy being around; the people you have the most fun with and positive connection to. Call, text or email them and set up some dates to spend time together, doing things that you enjoy. If you can't golf due to pain, do something else.

Summary

- Enjoyment is an effective antidote to pain.

- Reduce the impact of negative relationships; optimise the impact of positive ones.

- Play as much golf as the first two Rules of Rehabilitation permit.

15
Last Hole

In this chapter, I cover a few miscellaneous but important topics before heading for the conclusion at the nineteenth hole.

Bending forwards

Earlier I covered sitting and other postures, but one of the most frequent Triggers and Aggravators for LBP is bending forwards. Part of Prevention is also about performing Triggers and Aggravators differently, such that they are no longer working against you. Bending forwards was my most common Trigger, sometimes with load (lifting something), but usually a very light load. In our clinic, around 80% of LBP sufferers

PAIN-FREE AND CONFIDENT GOLF

find that sitting aggravates their pain. This is partly because most people bend forwards slightly in their lower backs when sitting, especially in a car.

If this doesn't apply to you, you may choose to ignore this practice. If your LBP is worse when you bend forwards, I highly recommend changing your movement patterns to a less triggering and more mechanically efficient and powerful way. Try the hip hinge.

The hip hinge

When you bend forwards (flexion), there are three areas that can contribute to that movement:

1. Your spine can bend.

2. Your hips can bend.

3. Your knees and ankles can bend.

Many people bend their spines first. If you have an unstable or weak spine, that's a bad idea. It makes much more sense to stabilise your spine, keeping it in neutral while the other parts do the work.

This should be easy for a golfer. Bend your hips first, and lightly brace your abdominal muscles while you do that. How to brace? Take a short sharp sniff through your nose – you'll feel your abdominal muscles tighten a bit. Hold that tightness while you hip hinge.

If you have done yoga or Pilates, you may struggle with this because it's likely you've been taught to roll up and down your spinal joints. If you are Flexion Intolerant – with or without instability – this is a bad idea. The hip hinge is covered in the Rapid Relief Plan (see Chapter 3 for QR code).

For many Flexion Intolerant LBP sufferers, this has been a game changer. Learn to hip hinge and make it your default movement pattern when you bend forwards. Remember, if bending forwards/flexion is a Trigger or Aggravator for you, and you're following the Rules of Rehabilitation, then you need to find another way of doing it. This is it.

Once you nail the hip hinge, you will progress to the hip hinge and squat, and from there to the hip hinge, squat and curl. This will give you a full range of movement in forward bending in a way that is maximally efficient and powerful. By following the rules, you can progress all the way to achieving your SMART goal. This is all covered in the supplementary online Rapid Relief Plan (see Chapter 3 for QR code).

How should you progress? You should have this by now. By following Rule of Rehabilitation 2: Start low and build slow (see Chapter 12).

Pre-game warm-up

If you're going to swing a club with enough speed to exert a force on your lower back – that's eight times your total body weight – don't you think it's worth warming up for that? By 'warm-up', I don't mean a bacon roll and a mug of coffee. Neither does three swings of your driver on the tee count – that's a great way of triggering an episode.

How do the pros warm up? They start with putting, then chipping with their wedge, and slowly move up the clubs to finish with the driver. Many pros will spend ninety minutes warming up. Surely you can manage more than three swings? Especially if it means a pain-free round.

There are many possible warm-up combinations, but remember to always stick to the Rules of Rehabilitation. When we work with golfers one-to-one we give them a warm-up that's tailored to them. Given that you have persistent/recurrent LBP/sciatica, the below routine is my best guess:

1. **Warm up your hips with standing hip rotations.** Bend one knee up towards your chest, bring the knee out and then bring it down to the ground in the centre. Do this four times and then reverse the direction. Repeat with the other hip.

2. **Warm up your mid-back and shoulders with sitting rotations to either side.** Twist as far as

you can comfortably left then right, four times each side.

3. **Do some standing back extensions.** Lean backwards with your hands in the small of your back.

4. **Windmill your arms forwards and backwards.** Each arm should rotate for twenty seconds in each direction.

5. **Turn your head to look over each shoulder.** Do this three times on each side.

6. **Start with chipping.** Then move up the clubs.

TOP TIP

Take at least ten minutes to warm up. The earlier in your day it is, the longer your warm-up should be.

You'll find the pre-game warm-up and hip hinging routine are available for free in the Golfer's Pain-Free & Confident Community. Go to https://golf.painfree-andconfident.com/book-reader or scan the QR code below for access and navigate to the community area.

Practice makes habit

In the late 1970s I was at a pro-celebrity golfing event at Gleneagles and witnessed an absolute peach of a shot. Lee Trevino played a wedge out of a deep bunker, 10 yards from the front edge of the green – probably 35 yards from the pin. The ball popped up, landed 5 yards onto the green, rolled the remaining 20 yards, hit the pin and dropped. Amid the applause, we heard a man call out, 'What a lucky shot!' Trevino came straight back with the line, 'Yeah, the more I practise, the luckier I get.' As a child, I didn't know that Gary Player was the first to deliver this line. This is totally relevant in achieving a long-term solution.

You're probably acquainted with the phrase 'practice makes perfect'. This is rarely true – few of us achieve true perfection in any field. The phrase 'practice makes habit' is much more on the money. As a committed golfer, you probably have lots of experience with this. It should come as no surprise to you that you have to put in the practice if you're going to keep taking steps back from the edge and achieve the goal of solving your pain and regaining your confidence.

The road to recovery isn't straight. It's twisting and turning with bumps. You will need to keep practising your Preventers and reducing your Risks. By doing this you will build healthier habits. Once you have established those habits, that's when it gets easy.

If you want to improve your golf, you have to practise. If you want to improve your back (so that you can play more golf for longer), you will also have to practise. I've given you six Essential Practices. You will have noticed that these are not separate practices; they are all connected and they complement one another. Just as your body and mind are connected, so are the practices. They are not discrete, they are integrated. You need to take this integrated, holistic approach to combat persistent pain. If you can find a way of mastering persistent pain and building a strong pain-free lower back without doing so, please let me know because I'd like to invest in that solution. You'll make billions.

Making several – or ideally all – of these practices a habit is the easiest way to get right back from the edge. How do you successfully build new habits and break unhelpful ones? I'm going to give you a crash course. Before I do, let's take a look at your swing.

Modifying your swing

As you might expect by now, any swing modifications should be seen through the lens of either Relief or Prevention. In the Relief phase, swing modifications should be about the reduce practice, ie reducing the aggravation of your pain. In the Prevention phase, swing modifications should be about the optimise practice, and relate to your long-term goal.

Relief phase

This is about reducing your pain. Ideally, this does not mean no golf.

- **Swing amplitude:** The obvious practice, which many golfers resist, is to reduce the size and speed of your backswing. This is likely to reduce the size and speed of your follow-through, thereby reducing the force on your lower back and resulting in less pain. Try it.

- **Change the forces by changing your set-up:** If you change your set-up, you will change the force distribution and dissipation. Many golfers find that by opening out their lead foot, it makes it easier to rotate through, thereby reducing the force on your lower back. If you have your feet closer together, it tends to result in less weight shifting going on, and therefore greater balance. That probably means less pain.

- **Step-through:** While the step-through helps you with weight transference, it also reduces the forces on your lower back. Try that too.

Prevention phase

In this phase you must be clear what you are optimising for. I don't just mean how many holes you want to play in a week. When you set a SMART goal, the 'A' stands for 'achievable'. It may not be achievable for you to play eighteen holes five days a week. When our team works with golfers this is something we spend a lot of time on at the outset, working out – based on many individual factors – what is likely to be achievable.

Broadly, the longer and more recently you've had pain, and the older and less fit you are, the fewer holes are achievable. It is vital that once you've set a goal that you are optimising for that goal. In this phase, the second Rule of Rehabilitation is more relevant and you should bear in mind Gabbett's ACWR (see Chapter 12). If you're a senior golfer, it is unlikely your body can deal with the forces it could when you were younger. You shouldn't try. Yes, you should keep trying to improve your capacity, but be realistic and don't break the second rule.

While you should be trying to get stronger as you age, there is a tension between this and your natural biological ageing. We all know that young adults are stronger than older adults. They are also more flexible. The strongest eighty-year-old is always weaker than the strongest forty-year-old. You should keep trying to optimise, but you should also ensure that your goal is achievable.

With this in mind, are there swing adaptations that will extend your longevity in golf? Yes, there are.

There are swings that are easier on most golfers' bodies than other swings. Below I list the pros and cons of the better-known swings:

- **The Classical Swing (Ben Hogan, Sam Snead):** This was popular before the 1980s and includes a full-body turn, with hips and shoulders rotating together. This reduces the torque and therefore the stress on the lower back. These 'olden day golfers' (I'm one) should last longer than those with a modern swing.

- **The X-Factor Swing (Tiger Woods and most current tour players):** This has been heavily used since the 1990s and encourages a separation between trunk and hip movement. This results in greater torque due to coiling the upper body in relation to the hips and legs and then releasing this with more force generated. Unfortunately, the lower back often suffers.

- **The Stack and Tilt Swing (Mike Weir):** This was developed in the early 2000s and encourages you to keep your weight on the forward/lead foot. It generally causes a more aggressive strike with often more compression on the facet joints in the lower back.

- **The Single Plane Swing (Bryson DeChambeau – adapted version):** This keeps the club and arms in a single plane, with more wrist and shoulder movement. It reduces force on the

lower back, but increases the risk of wrist and
shoulder strain.

To summarise, the Classical Swing and Single Plane
Swing are gentler on the lower back; the X-Factor
Swing and Stack and Tilt Swing put more strain on
the lumbar spine. Beyond the above, there are many
possible modifications, and the best ones for you will
depend on your unique physical capacities. Yes, I'm
saying you should – if you can afford it – have an
analysis of your physical capacity.

Putting

Most golfers are pretty good at bending at the hips
and keeping their lower back in neutral when playing
woods and irons. When you putt, do you bend your
lower back rather than your hips? If you crouch over
your putts, you'll be bending your lower back. If you
are Flexion Intolerant, my advice would be not to do
that – at least, not during the Relief phase.

Here in my own backyard, in East Lothian, Scotland,
former European PGA golf coach Gary Nicol has an
interesting approach to the swing too. Gary Nicol has
coached over thirty European Tour professionals and
numerous Ryder Cup players. He's coached at all the
Majors. When I met Gary, he asked me: 'When you
were first taught to play golf, were you taught to pull

through with your lead arm or push through with your trail arm?'

I'm right-handed, so my trail hand is my right. Like everyone I knew, I'd been taught to pull through with my left. Gary pointed out that this is the equivalent of being a tennis player trying to play a backhand shot with the weaker, less-coordinated hand. Why would you do that? Following his guidance, I focused on pushing gently with my right. Bingo; it was so much easier. It's amazing to me how seemingly subtle changes have what feels like global impacts on ease of swing.

I know I've mentioned this before, but it's worth repeating. Gary taught me to breathe out during my downswing. I had no idea I was holding my breath when swinging. Holding your breath causes quite a lot of tension and that's bad for pain and for performance.

TRY IT YOURSELF

Breathe out on the downswing.

Because the golf swing is often an Aggravator, we include swing analysis and coaching in our Accelerator programme. If you're wondering what on earth to do with your swing – short- and long-term – you only have to ask. See our Pain-Free & Confident Accelerator (flick to Chapter 16 for the QR code).

Change your habits

Playing your ball to the right position for the next shot is crucial in golf. It's the same with habit changing; you have to set yourself up for success. When you find yourself in a difficult lie, it's because the last shot didn't go well.

How can you set yourself up well for making sure you succeed every day? Here comes a crash course in habit changing. Again, I'm standing on the shoulders of giants – such as BJ Fogg, Sunstein and Thaler, James Clear, Stephen Guise and others. If you've read any of their works, you will see much of it reflected here. To be fair, I had worked out quite a bit of this stuff through my own failures in my twenties. They have published research papers and books on the subject – many of which I have read and incorporated into my own approach to habit change. It's important that I recognise and credit their contribution to my approach. Systemising for habit change is vital – as mentioned in Chapter 3, your motivation dips as your pain lessens. You have to put the ball in the right position for your next shot.

What will you actually do daily, ie which habit will you choose to work on? Ideally start with one. Once you've got a few weeks of momentum, perhaps add another (remember SLABS?). You might choose the easiest or you might choose the one you think will have the greatest impact. Your selection can be made from the six Essential Practices.

Prompts

If you want to make hip hinging a habit, practise it every time you do something you do every day, such as brushing your teeth. Use these or other prompts to remind you to practise your new habit.

> **TRY IT YOURSELF**
>
> Especially if you are Flexion Intolerant, practise hip hinging every time you brush your teeth, wash or dry your hands, or prepare food in the kitchen. Use these activities to act as prompts to do the behaviour. The more often you practise hip hinging, the more you will groove that movement pattern.

Habit stacking

When you finish brushing your teeth and hip hinging then get down on the floor and do some Preventer exercises. That way you are stacking one good habit on top of another. You can build this up into a long virtuous cycle.

Habit levels

I credit Stephen Guise (2019) in particular here, and highly recommend his book *Elastic Habits*. This was definitely his idea rather than one I developed myself.

He calls it a habit grid. The idea is that it is vital to maintain momentum with habit changing. As Guise says, in order not to miss a day, it helps to have a low-effort habit. Ideally when trying to establish a habit, you don't want to miss two days in a row. One is excusable, as you can recover from one lost day.

Guise recommends having three levels for any habit – an entry level, intermediate level and advanced level. I call these 'got it', 'nailed it' and 'smashed it' because these terms have celebration built into them:

- 'Got it' is easy to achieve.

- 'Nailed it' is more challenging.

- 'Smashed it' is stretching yourself.

Below, I offer some examples of habit grids. You must create your own, as these examples may not be remotely similar to your own personal practices. This should give you a framework that you can then popu-late with your own ideas and start applying.

Here's one showing physical activity.

Physical activity

Optimise physical activity	Got it	Nailed it	Smashed it
Walk/run	Walk a mile	Walk/run a mile	Run a mile
Steps	3,000 per day	7,000 per day	10,000 per day
Push-ups	1 a day	10 a day	40 a day

Here's another for nutrition.

Nutrition

Optimise nutrition	Got it	Nailed it	Smashed it
Time-restricted feeding	Only eat between 7am and 8pm	Only eat between 7am and 6pm	Only eat between 10am and 8pm
Snacking	Maximum 2 snacks per day	Maximum 1 snack per day	No snacks between meals
Vegetable consumption	3 handfuls a day	5 handfuls a day	7 handfuls a day

You get the idea? The 'got it' level has to be so easy that you won't fail to do it. Therefore, on a given day in this example you will have one 'got it' – let's say walk a mile. You might have three levels: a 'got it', a 'nailed it' and a 'smashed it'. There are many possibilities. Whatever happens, you'll have done at least something to keep your momentum going.

Here's one for sleep.

Sleep

Optimise sleep	Got it	Nailed it	Smashed it
Stop work time	9pm	8pm	7pm
Read fiction before lights go out	2 minutes	10 minutes	30 minutes
Get daylight	2 minutes by 10am	5 minutes by 9am	15 minutes by 9am

The possibilities are endless. You have the framework.

TRY IT YOURSELF

Take thirty to sixty minutes to draw up your habit grid and fill in the blanks. Remember your 'got it' has to be easy peasy – make sure it's totally doable; that way you won't miss a day.

Tracking changes by keeping score

One useful tool in maintaining your momentum is to be able to see it. We're all motivated by positive feedback. You have a scorecard in golf, and it's helpful to have one in habit changing too. Get yourself a calendar – I prefer good old paper ones for this, but you could do it digitally (even just using a spreadsheet). At the end of each day, mark on the calendar a score for that day.

Here is Stephen Guise's scoring system:

- One 'got it' = one point
- One 'nailed it' = two points
- One 'smashed it' = three points

It's perfectly possible to have more than one point, depending on how many habits you're tracking and what level you've achieved in that habit. You should never have a zero day – because your 'got its' are so easy that you're not going to miss a day. Even if the cat dies, you lose your job and your favourite team gets relegated – you will still have at least one 'got it' that day – every day you are winning, and making progress towards your goal. Give yourself a pat on the back and keep practising.

There are many more tactics, especially when it comes to breaking bad habits. My other favourite book in this genre is James Clear's *Atomic Habits* (2018). Here are some ways to break a bad habit, based on Clear's insights:

- Put the trigger out of sight.
- Make it less appealing to do.
- Make it harder to do.
- Make it less rewarding to do.

Although this section on habit changing is brief, it's all that most people will need. I highly recommend the books cited above for a fuller understanding of this important topic.

Summary

- Hip hinging is a useful approach to bending forwards.

- The warm-up is essential for optimising.

- There are many ways of modifying your swing to reduce load and optimise performance.

- Habit change is hard, but there are some well-proven frameworks.

16

Conclusion At The Nineteenth Hole

I n this final chapter, we wrap up all that you've learnt and focus on applying that learning.

You have your course map (the Cliff of Pain), you have three Rules of Rehabilitation to play by, you have your six Essential Practices, and now you know how to establish a new habit and break a bad one.

I separate the Relief phase from the Prevention phase to demonstrate that they are different processes, but, in practice, if you have had pain for years, I have found that you have to tackle both simultaneously. This is due to the complexity of pain. It's so easy to relapse with persistent pain that the two stages must usually be played together. It's like driving and putting all in one.

There's also a learning phase in this process. You have to experiment. The quickest way to learn is by making mistakes – I hope they aren't too painful. By learning from your mistakes, you will be a little wiser. As a guide, the longer you have had pain, the longer this learning period lasts. Stick with it. You will make progress if you follow the process outlined in this book.

TOP TIP

Please go back, read the book again and make notes – take your time over this. Before you start again, put the book down and review what you've learnt.

Consider this question: 'How important is it for you to have a strong pain-free lower back you can have confidence in?' If it's important, then bring your attention to focus on this goal. Knowledge is not enough. You have to do the work. All that stands between you and becoming a golfer who has a strong pain-free lower back you can have confidence in is practice. As Jack Nicklaus would say: 'Do the work.'

Playing out of bunkers

Another way to think about learning from your mistakes is that the Cliff of Pain is littered with bunkers – don't be put off by these. Again, due to complexity, it's highly likely you will land in a bunker, but it's the trend that's important.

How do you know what the trend is? Track your Backscore (see Chapter 9).

If you need to play backwards out of a bunker before moving forwards, then do that. Remember that over-all you're making progress. Mistakes happen. Notice them and move on. It's the next shot that matters.

A winning future

If you apply the frameworks you have read about in this book, you will optimise your chances of mas-tering your LBP or sciatica, just as I did and just as thousands of other long-term sufferers have done. As I said at the beginning, it's not easy but it is simple – stick to the plan.

You don't have to do this alone. LBP affects 80% of golfers at some time in their lives, while sciatica affects around 20%. If you want to put a group together, either at your golf club or your workplace, I often give talks on this framework. If you throw in a round of golf, I'd love to come and visit your club or place of work. You can reach me through: info@painfreeand-confident.com

Remember, we run **free workshops** fortnightly; go to https://golf.painfreeandconfident.com/workshop or scan the QR code below:

For a **Rapid Relief Plan**, prevention exercises and group support by the Active X Clinical Team, go to http://golf.painfreeandconfident.com/book-reader or scan the QR code below:

There's also our 16-week **Pain-free & Confident Accelerator** programme, if you want to optimise your chances of getting right back from the edge: visit https://golf.painfreeandconfident.com/pac-program or scan the QR code below:

If you haven't got your Pain-free and Confident score-card yet, or if you did it earlier and would like to see how much you've learnt or put into practice, get it here: https://go.painfreeandconfident.com

I hope to see you on the course, getting right back from the edge and building your strong, pain-free lower back you can have confidence in.

Summary

- You have the plan you needed.

- You can only succeed if you prioritise and apply the knowledge.

- There is often a learning phase – this takes more time the longer you've had your pain.

- You will land in bunkers and may have to play backwards in order to progress.

- There are many free resources open to you as a reader of this book.

Bibliography

Brinjikji, W. *et al.* (2015) 'Systematic literature review of imaging features of spinal degeneration in asymptomatic populations', *American Journal of Neuroradiology*, 36(4), 811–816. Available at: https://doi.org/10.3174/ajnr.A4173

Chaparro, L.E., Furlan, A.D., Deshpande, A. *et al.* (2013) 'Opioids compared to placebo or other treatments for chronic low-back pain', *Cochrane Database of Systematic Reviews*, 8. Available at: https://doi.org/10.1002/14651858.CD004959.pub4

Chapman, C.R., Tuckett, R.P. and Song, C.W. (2008) 'Pain and stress in a systems perspective: Reciprocal neural, endocrine, and immune interactions', *The Journal of Pain*, 9(2), 122–145. Available at: https://doi.org/10.1016/j.jpain.2007.09.006

Clear, J. (2018) *Atomic Habits*. London: Penguin.

Cook, E. (2024) 'Ouch! Solving the riddle of pain', *The Guardian* (22 December). Available at: www.theguardian.com/lifeandstyle/2024/dec/22/ouch-solving-the-riddle-of-pain

Da Silva, T., Mills, K., Brown, B.T. *et al.* (2019) 'Recurrence of low back pain is common: A prospective inception cohort study', *Journal of Physiotherapy*, 65(3), 159–165. Available at: www.sciencedirect.com/science/article/pii/S1836955319300591#cebib0010

Engel, G.L. (1977) 'The need for a new medical model: A challenge for biomedicine', *Science*, 196(4286), 129–136. Available at: https://doi.org/10.1126/science.847460

Finan, P.H., Goodin, B.R. and Smith, M.T. (2013) 'The association of sleep and pain: An update and a path forward', *The Journal of Pain*, 14(12), 1539–1552. Available at: https://doi.org/10.1016/j.jpain.2013.08.007

Fisher, J.P., Hassan, D.T. and O'Connor, N. (1995) 'Minerva', *The British Medical Journal*, 310(70). Available at: https://doi.org/10.1136/bmj.310.6971.70

Gabbett, T.J. (2016) 'The training–injury prevention paradox: Should athletes be training smarter and harder?', *British Journal of Sports Medicine*, 50(5), 273–280. Available at: https://doi.org/10.1136/bjsports-2015-095788

Gabbett, T.J. (2020) 'Debunking the myths about training load, injury and performance: Empirical evidence, hot topics and recommendations for practitioners', *British Journal of Sports Medicine*, 54(1), 58–66. Available at: www.researchgate. net/publication/328544835_Debunking_the_ myths_about_training_load_injury_and_ performance_Empirical_evidence_hot_topics_and_ recommendations_for_practitioners

Guise, S. (2019) *Elastic Habits: How to create smarter habits that adapt to your day*. Orlando: Selective Entertainment LLC.

Hosea, T.M., Gatt, C.J. and Galli, K.M. (2010) 'Biomechanical analysis of the golfer's back', in A.J. Cochran (ed.) *Science and Golf (Routledge Revivals)*. Abingdon: Taylor & Francis. Available at: http:// ebookcentral.proquest.com

Jocko, 'Episode 427: Work Hard and Be Useful: With Arnold Schwarzenegger', Jocko Podcast (2024). Available at: https://jockopodcast. com/2024/02/28/427-work-hard-and-be-useful- with-arnold-schwarzenegger

Kim, S.H., Park, J.Y. and Shin, H.E. *et al.* (2019) 'The influence of rapid eye movement sleep deprivation on nociceptive transmission and the duration of facial allodynia in rats: A behavioral and Fos immunohistochemical study', *The Journal of Headache and Pain*, 20(21). Available at: https://doi. org/10.1186/s10194-019-0977-0

Lethem, J., Slade, P.D., Troup, J.D.G. *et al.* (1983) 'Outline of a fear-avoidance model of exaggerated pain perception—I', *Behaviour Research and Therapy*, 21(4), 401–408. Available at: https://doi.org/10.1016/0005-7967(83)90009-8

Lorimer Moseley, G. and Butler, D.S. (2015) 'Fifteen years of explaining pain: The past, present, and future',*The Journal of Pain*, 16(9), 807–813. Available at: https://doi.org/10.1016/j.jpain.2015.05.005

Melzack, R. and Wall, P.D. (1965) 'Pain mechanisms: A new theory', *Science*, 150(3699), 971–979. Available at: https://doi.org/10.1126/science.150.3699.971

Roland, M. and Morris, R.W. (1983) 'A study of the natural history of back pain. Part 1: Development of a reliable and sensitive measure of disability in low back pain', *Spine*, 8(2), 141–144. Available at: https://doi.org/10.1097/00007632-198303000-00004

Schon, K.R., Parker, A.P.J. and Woods, C.G. (2018) *Congenital Insensitivity to Pain Overview*. Seattle: University of Washington. Available at: https://europepmc.org/article/nbk/nbk481553

Shimo, K., Uneo, T., Younger, J. *et al.* (2011) 'Visualization of painful experiences believed to trigger the activation of affective and emotional brain regions in subjects with low back pain', *PLOS ONE*, 6(11). Available at: https://doi.org/10.1371/journal.pone.0026681

Somma, F., Negro, A., D'Agostino, V. *et al.* (2022) 'COVID-19 and low back pain: Previous infections lengthen recovery time after intradiscal ozone therapy in patients with herniated lumbar disc', *La Radiologia Medica*, 127(6), 673–680. Available at: https://doi.org/10.1007/s11547-022-01500-w

Su, B. and O'Connor, J.P. (2013) 'NSAID therapy effects on healing of bone, tendon, and the enthesis', *Journal of Applied Physiology*, 115(6), 892–899. Available at: https://doi.org/10.1152/japplphysiol.00053.2013

The Lancet (2023) 'The global epidemic of low back pain', *The Lancet* (Vol 5, June). Available at: www.thelancet.com/pdfs/journals/lanrhe/PIIS2665-9913(23)00133-9.pdf

Titleist Performance Institute (n.d.) *The Golfer's Guide to Lower Back Pain – Part 1*. Available at: www.mytpi.com/articles/health/the-golfer's-guide-to-lower-back-pain-part-1

World Health Organization (2020) *Global Burden of Disease Study*. Available at: www.who.int/data/global-health-estimates

Acknowledgements

The world of pain research is rich and evolving. In writing this book I have been standing on the shoulders of giants. The Master's degree I gained gave me the time to dive deep – but it also taught me humility. There is so much to learn and it keeps evolving. I'd like to credit the tutors – especially Dr Sarah Henderson – teaching the MSc in The Clinical Management of Pain at The University of Edinburgh www.ed.ac.uk/clinical-sciences/pain-management. Another academic source of continued learning for me has been The NOI Group in Australia: www.noigroup.com.

Thank you to the thousands of patients who have put their trust in me – golfers and non-golfers alike. It is a privilege to have helped you. I'm only sorry that early in my career I was not always successful in helping

221

people to overcome pain, but every failure has taught me something. Collectively, they have all taught me to stay curious, to remember Doc Randall's advice and to keep striving to get better.

My family have also inspired me to improve. I thank my wife Natasha for affording me the time to work on this book, and all the long hours I have spent in the clinic. Without her support at home and in my work, I could not have achieved all that I have. As a past fellow sciatica sufferer, she had plenty of insights too. Thank you to my Mum Val for her never-ending interest and encouragement. Thanks go to my brother Alistair and his wife Nikki in supporting my work recently.

Thank you to my golfing buddies, who continue to invite me to play, despite my lack of practice and consequent failure to improve. You're right – I haven't prioritised my golf for a long time, but I do enjoy playing.

A huge thanks to Michael Basoco, Andrew Neil, Robin Stewart and Ken Massie for their generosity in reading my first draft and providing invaluable feedback. This book would have been a mess of ideas with a distinct lack of structure without your suggestions and corrections.

Thank you to Daniel Priestley and the team at Dent Global. Their mentoring gave me the confidence to push the 'go' button to start writing this book.

Finally, thank you to the team at Rethink Press for putting their trust in me and bringing this book to you.

I'm glad I've written it. I hope you are too. Thank you for taking the time to read all the way to the end. It's that sort of thoroughness that will help you to achieve a long-term solution.

The Author

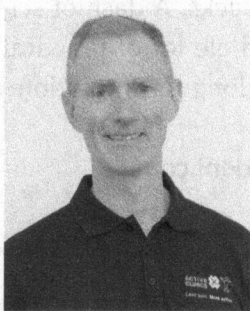

Gavin Routledge is a Gold Medallist from the British School of Osteopathy (1991) and a lifelong student of pain. Having specialised in lower back pain and sciatica for over three decades, Gavin is also a certified health coach and lifestyle medicine professional. He combines clinical expertise with a deep passion for golf, sparked at the age of nine while watching pro-celebrity matches at Gleneagles, where he promptly fell in love with the game. His grandfather gave him his first set of (ladies') clubs, and he was off.

After enduring seven years of his own back pain and sciatica in his twenties, Gavin finally reached a tipping point. He decided it was time to master his own lower back. He did exactly that, then went on to write *The Back Book* (HarperCollins, 1997), followed by a Master's in Pain Management from The University of Edinburgh in 2012, and a second book on lower back pain in 2017.

Now, with thirty-four years in clinical practice and thousands of relieved backs to his name, Gavin brings a golfer's heart and a clinician's mind to his latest work. What's his mission? To help fellow golf lovers stay on the course – and out of the chiropractor's office – by showing them how to relieve pain and then rebuild strength and confidence in their backs. A dash of science, a dose of humour and a whole lot of practical help – this book is your route to a long-term solution.

🌐 https://golf.painfreeandconfident.com

f www.facebook.com/activexbacks

in www.linkedin.com/in/gavinroutledge

◎ www.instagram.com/activexbacks

www.ingramcontent.com/pod-product-compliance
Lightning Source LLC
Chambersburg PA
CBHW010113270326
41927CB00018B/3369